Bovine Meat Inspection

Anatomy, physiol[illegible]

Bovine Meat Inspection

Anatomy, physiology and disease conditions

A Grist

NOTTINGHAM
University Press

Nottingham University Press
Manor Farm, Main Street, Thrumpton
Nottingham NG11 0AX, United Kingdom
www.nup.com

NOTTINGHAM

First published 2005

British Library Cataloguing in Publication Data
Bovine Meat Inspection
Anatomy, physiology and disease conditions:
A Grist

ISBN 1-904761-75-5

Disclaimer

Every reasonable effort has been made to ensure that the material in this book is true, correct, complete and appropriate at the time of writing. Nevertheless, the publishers and authors do not accept responsibility for any omission or error, or for any injury, damage, loss or financial consequences arising from the use of the book.

Typeset by Nottingham University Press, Nottingham
Printed and bound by Hobbs the Printers, Hampshire, England

INTRODUCTION

This book has been designed to provide a study aid for students undertaking the Royal Society for the Promotion of Health Red Meat Inspection Certificate and other courses where knowledge of bovine meat inspection is required such as those for Environmental Health Officers and Official Veterinary Surgeons

It is hoped that it may also provide information in a 'user friendly' format for abattoir owners and producers as to the nature of rejections recorded by inspectors.

Wherever possible, photographs illustrating anatomical features and conditions have been included, the latter generally depicting severe examples of conditions. This is a conscious decision, arrived at after giving numerous lectures on meat inspection where I learnt that no two people would describe something the same way.

The section covering anatomy and physiology does not go into great detail; numerous other texts fulfil this function. The order that the bodily systems are introduced should not be construed as an order of importance.

The section covering diseases loosely follows the format of name, synonym, aetiology, pathogenesis, clinical lesions, gross lesions and judgement as to the fitness for human consumption. The diseases are listed in alphabetical order for ease of reference.

The affections of specific parts and conditions encountered at post-mortem inspection in abattoirs were added to the original manuscript as it was felt they would provide a useful tool for day-to-day inspection decisions in the abattoir environment.

AUTHOR DISCLAIMER

I must add that the judgements as to the fitness for human consumption given in this book are my own views, gained through experience and consultation with others.

A Grist

ACKNOWLEDGEMENTS

Acknowledging the assistance given to an author in preparing a book is customary and in my view should be given greater status. This book would not have been possible without the patience and assistance given by the following people:

William (Bill) Boxall, for his encouragement and belief.

Martin Wood BA MSc FCIEH, Tim Udall MRCVS and Rita Hinton of the Langford School of Veterinary Science, for teaching their students that they can and should try to make a difference. I hope this book can be considered as part repayment for their efforts.

Alison Small BVM&S DVPH(MH) MRCVS of the Division of Food Animal Science, Bristol University for supplying encouragement, photographs and advice, and the support of Ian McKirgan and Martin Evans of the Meat Hygiene Service.

Thanks are due to the following Meat Hygiene Inspectors: Colin Walters, who taught me how to take photographs, Fiona Whalley, Gordon Gait, Julian Ponting, Eric Harvey and Grace Grist but mostly to Dave Barrah, for providing photographs, information, enthusiasm, support and knowledge.

The following abattoirs allowed photographs of anatomy to be taken, despite the time and occasional delays my presence caused: F. Drury and Sons, Tockenham, Wiltshire, and C and S Meats, Holness, Sherborne, Dorset. Thanks go to the management and production staff of these establishments especially Dave Tipper and the slaughtermen at F. Drury and Sons.

Ben Lacey MA VetMB MRCVS veterinary adviser for Pfizer Animal Health for supplying some photographs of parasitic conditions and Manuel Sarnago MRCVS for supplying photographs and advice on other conditions.

My children, George, Elizabeth and Henry, who not only gave encouragement but also edited and labelled pictures, illustrating once again that they are far more confident in the use of computers than their father.

The patience of Nottingham University Press and especially Sarah Keeling cannot be emphasised enough. As with the poultry inspection book, she fielded panic phone calls and alterations with a calm manner that put me to shame.

Most gratitude must go to my wife, Grace, who as a practicing Meat Hygiene Inspector offered support, patience, guidance, research assistance, editorial support and a grasp of the English Language that has become my safety net.

DEDICATION

I have always held the opinion, during my time as a Meat Hygiene Inspector, abattoir manager and lecturer that the food that I inspect should be fit for my own children to eat. If you would not feed it to your own children, you should not expect the consumer to feed it to theirs.

To that end I dedicate this to my wife Grace and my children George, Elizabeth, Henry and Harriette.

CONTENTS

DIAGRAM LIST

PHOTOGRAPH LIST

Page

Section One
Anatomy

Section Two
Diseases

Section Three
Parasites

Section Four
Neoplasia

Section Five
Conditions Encountered at Post Mortem Inspection in Abattoirs

Section Six
Anatomy Aide Memoire

Photograph list

[1] Author's own photographs
[2] Courtesy of Mr David Barrah
[3] Courtesy of Mr Eric Harvey
[4] Courtesy of Miss Alison Small BVM&S DVPH(MH) MRCVS
[5] Courtesy of Mr Manuel Sarnago MRCVS
[6] Courtesy of Mr Ben Lacey MA VetMB MRCVS
[7] Courtesy of Mr Colin Walters

FOREWORD

Andy Grist's first textbook in this series, Poultry Inspection, provided a much needed guide for trainee meat inspectors, plant inspection assistants and veterinary surgeons working in the poultry industry. This second book, Bovine Meat Inspection, fulfils a similar role and by focussing on one species rationalises the learning process. The text follows a logical progression of basic anatomy and physiology and then leads into the disease process by cause and effect. Each condition is described and clearly illustrated and includes the decision making process as to fitness for human consumption. Sections on conditions affecting specific parts of bovines and commonly encountered post mortem conditions are of particularly practical use in the abattoir and an 'aide memoire' provides excellent revision material.

Changes in legislation throughout Europe, in the whole of the food chain, gives additional importance to Andy's series of meat inspection guides. All Official Veterinarians and Official Auxiliaries (which the UK will continue to describe as Meat Hygiene Inspectors) will require to have achieved proscribed levels of competence and have passed examinations to prove it. Andy's book provides the basic information necessary to achieve the competence required in post-mortem inspection of cattle.

Beef has been restored to its rightful place as the main red meat eaten in the United Kingdom. The dedication of the inspection team has done much to restore consumers' confidence that the meat they eat, having been inspected by professionals, is safe and wholesome. I commend this book, produced by a member of that team. Students of meat inspection, qualified inspectors and meat plant operators will find this book invaluable for learning, revision, reference and teaching.

Tim Udall OBE BVSc CertVPH(MH) MRCVS
17 April 2005

1

ANATOMY/ PHYSIOLOGY

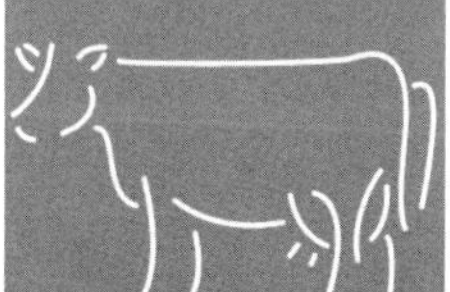

SKELETAL SYSTEM

INTRODUCTION

The skeletal system, the bones, provides structure, protection and a means of locomotion. Muscles are attached to the bones by ligaments or tendons and move the animal by contracting around a pivot or joint. In this section the basic structure, position and function of the bones is described. For this purpose the bones of the skeleton are divided into the skull, the axial skeleton and the appendicular skeleton (forelegs and hindlegs).

THE STRUCTURE OF BONES

Bone is a collagen matrix containing mineral salts, chiefly calcium phosphate, and various cells including osteoclasts and osteoblasts. The deposition of mineral salts within the matrix is controlled by osteoblasts. Mineral reabsorbtion and release of the minerals into the blood is attributed to the large, mononucleated osteoclasts. These cells work in balance, their activity being controlled by parathyroid hormone (PTH) secreted by the parathyroid gland in response to fluctuation in the serum- calcium level of the blood. If this level decreases more hormone is released which has the effect of increasing the activity of the osteoclasts whilst decreasing the osteoblast activity and hence subsequently increasing the calcium in the blood. This deposition and reabsorbtion of mineral salts of the bone is a continual process.

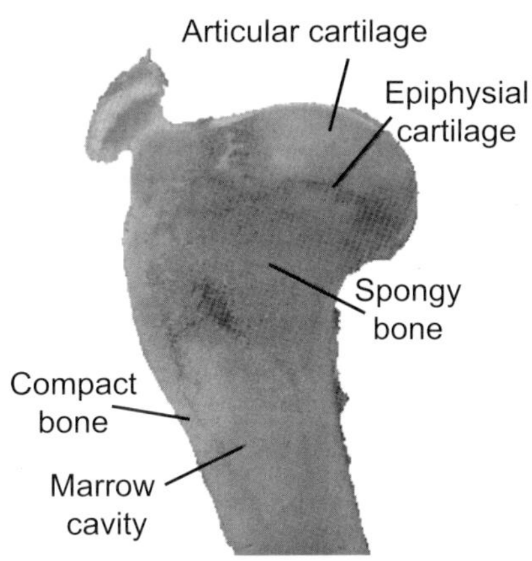

Longitudinal section of a bovine humerus

Bones have a connective tissue membranous covering, the periosteum, which has bone-forming properties and, through fusion with muscular connective tissue, anchors the muscle to the bone. Under the periosteum is the dense, or compact bone, which in the long bones forms a hollow shaft containing marrow and spongy bone. Marrow occurs in two forms, red and yellow, and is a combination of blood vessels and connective tissue containing fat and blood producing cells. Red marrow produces blood cells such as erythrocytes and leukocytes; yellow marrow is formed mainly from fatty tissue. Spongy or cancellous bone is usually found at the extremities of long bones and is composed of thin intersecting layers of bone. The articular cartilage has a bluish white colour and is also known as hyaline cartilage due to its glassy appearance. The epiphyseal cartilage represents the site at which bone growth increases the length of the long bones.

BONE TYPES

There are several classification systems used to describe bone types, the most common being the subdivision of bones into shapes, therefore the types encountered can be considered to be:

- Long bones, such as those of the humerus and femur.
- Short bones, such as the carpus and tarsus, roughly cuboid in shape.
- Flat bones, consisting of two layers of compact bone separated by a thin layer of spongy bone, as occurs in cranial bones and the scapula.
- Irregular bones, for example the vertebrae.

The body also contains a number of visceral bones, such as the *os calcis* that occurs in the bovine heart.

THE STRUCTURE OF JOINTS

The separate bones of the skeletal system are jointed together by systems that either fix the bone in relation to its neighbour or allow partial or free movement (articulation). Fibrous and cartilaginous joints between bones form fused or limited mobility joints, and synovial joints allow free movement between articulating bones.

Cartilaginous joints are found in areas such as between the vertebrae, at the pelvic symphysis and between the two halves of the mandible. Their structures vary and allow a small range of movement between the bones.

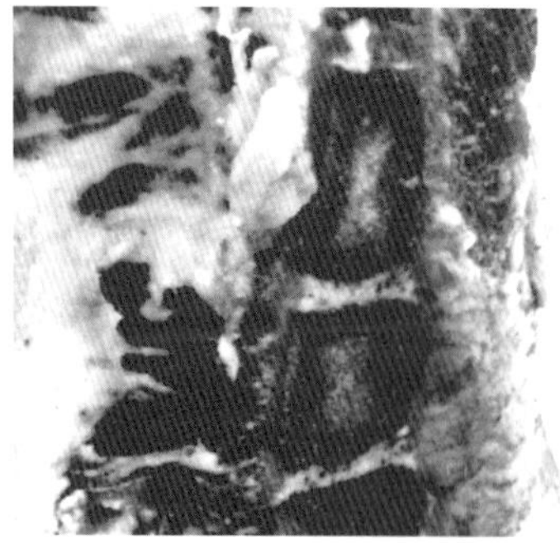

Cartilaginous joints in the sternum

Fibrous joints immobily connect bones forming joints such as those fusing the flat bones of the skull at joints known as sutures.

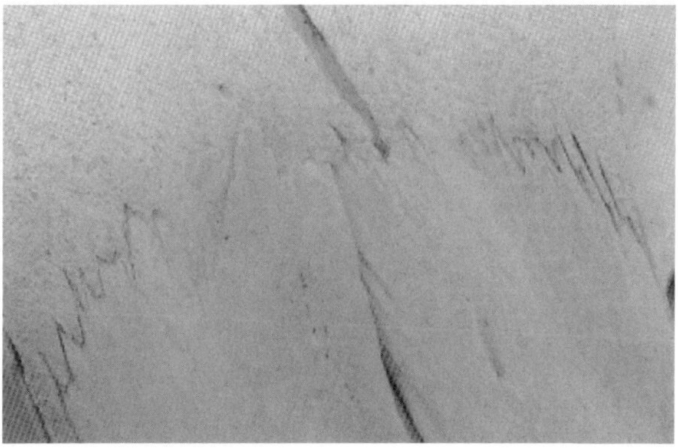

Sutures between flat bones of the skull

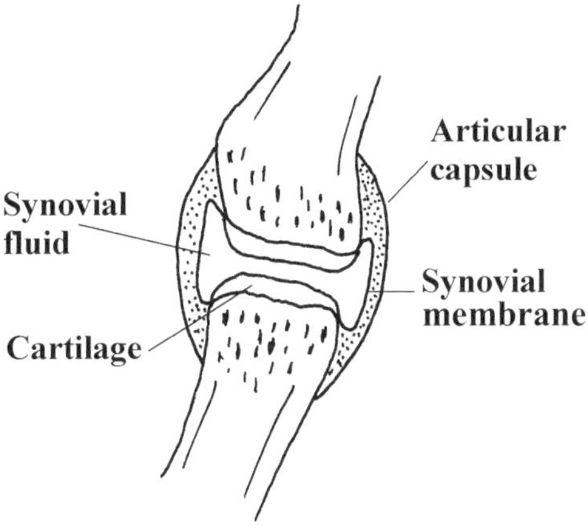

Synovial joints occur wherever free movement is required. The direction of movement (be it rotational or in one or two planes) is dependant on the structure of the articulating surface of the bones connected and the direction of the action of muscular activity. Synovial joints are mostly associated with the appendicular skeleton. The area of the joint is surrounded by a capsule (articular capsule) the inner surface of which consists of a membrane (synovial membrane). The articular capsule contains synovial fluid, a plasma-like fluid secreted by the synovial membrane that lubricates moving parts and nourishes the cartilage.

The pivoting plane of the joint is determined by the shape of the bones of the joint and the arrangement of the surrounding ligaments. This plane has been used to classify the various types of synovial joint into groups, two of which include the hinge joint of the elbow which provides for pendulum movement in one plane and the spheroidal joint (ball and socket) of the hip which allows both pendulum movement and a degree of rotation.

THE SKULL

The skull is formed from flat bones protecting the brain, formed by the cranium, facial bones and the lower jaw.

Fused joints called sutures, forming a dome within the cavity of which the brain is protected, join the cranial bones.

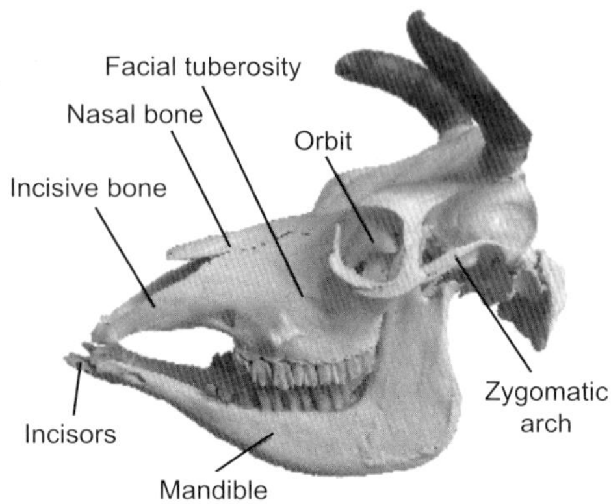

The facial bones, including the incisive and nasal bones, are again joined by sutures and house the organs of sight and smell. The nasal or turbinate bones form passageways or sinuses within the facial bones.

The lower jaw, the mandible, is U-shaped and very strong, capable of resisting the tremendous force exerted on it during the process of chewing. The entire mandible is made up of two halves, jointed at the chin by a mandibular symphysis, allowing a flexibility of rotation. The jaw is chiefly raised and lowered by the masseter muscles that are fused to the periosteum at the facial tuberosity.

THE AXIAL SKELETON

This term denotes the bones of the spine, the ribs and the pelvic girdle. The bones that comprise the spine are grouped together according to their position and function. The vertebrae are examples of irregular bones; they have small and irregular processes (projections) emanating from their dorsal and ventral surfaces. They have a central tunnel or canal which, when grouped with the other vertebrae form the spinal channel through which the spinal cord runs. The articulation between the vertebrae is of a semi mobile cartilaginous symphysis, allowing a small range of movement per vertebrae, but when taken as a whole allowing strength and flexibility of the spine.

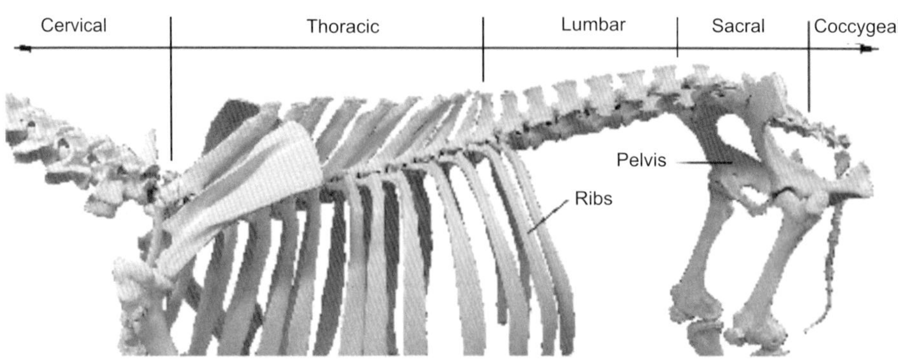

There are seven cervical vertebrae, (the skull articulating with the 1st cervical vertebrae, the axis bone), twelve to thirteen thoracic vertebrae (articulating with the ribs), six lumbar vertebrae (forming the roof of the abdominal cavity), five sacral vertebrae (fused together to form the synsacrum) and eighteen to twenty coccygeal or tail vertebrae.

THE RIBS

The bovine skeleton contains thirteen pairs of ribs articulating dorsally with the thoracic vertebrae. The ribs are classified by their relationship to the sternum, those that articulate ventrally with the sternum are known as true ribs, and those that do not are termed false ribs. The cavity formed by the thoracic vertebrae, ribs and sternum is the thorax.

THE PELVIS

The pelvis forms a cavity within the body. The roof of the cavity is formed by the fused sacral vertebrae, the sides and base by the right and left *os coxae* (the pelvic bones, a fusion of the ilium, ischium and pubis). The pelvic bones are joined posterially by the pelvic symphysis. The articular surface of the femur joins the pelvis at the acetabulum forming a ball and socket joint.

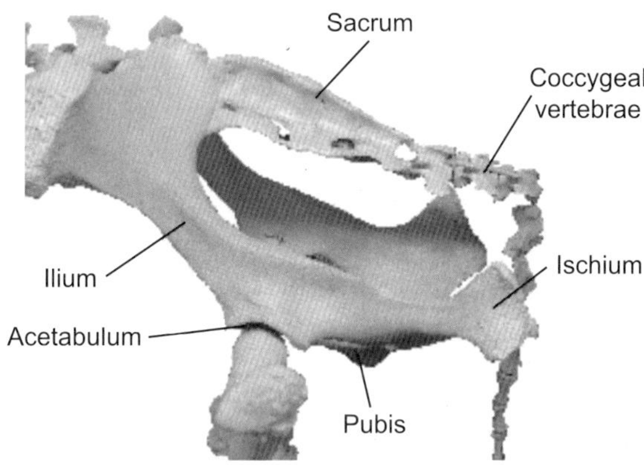

THE APPENDICULAR SKELETON

FORELEG

The foreleg is similar in nomenclature to the human arm. The scapula (shoulder blade) is held in position by muscle and connective tissue, and as such does not articulate with the axial skeleton proper. It is classed as a flat bone, triangular in shape with a surface spine. This bone terminates at a ball and socket joint at which point it articulates with the humerus.

The humerus is an example of a long bone, basically consisting of a hollow cylinder of dense bone surrounding marrow, as such it possesses great load bearing ability in the vertical plane. The proximal humerus has several projections of bone (tuberosities) that represent the point of attachment of musculature, including the greater tuberosity that forms the point of the shoulder.

Distally the humerus articulates with a hinge type synovial joint with the radius and ulna. In cattle the ulna is fused to the larger radius and extends to form the olecranon or elbow.

The carpus (wrist) is made up of six bones, articulating dorsally with the radius and ventrally with the metacarpus. The bones of the foot (phalanges) form two digits separated by an interdigital cleft that is prevented from splaying by interdigital ligaments in the live animal. It is worth noting that only the hooves proper are separated by the cleft.

Bovine foreleg

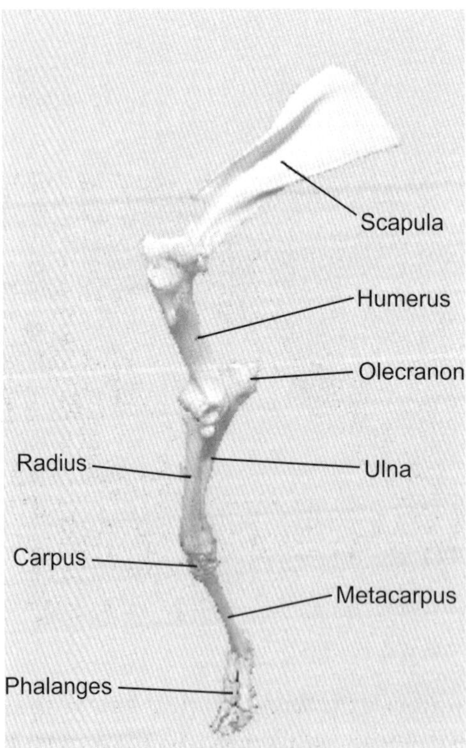

Bovine hindleg

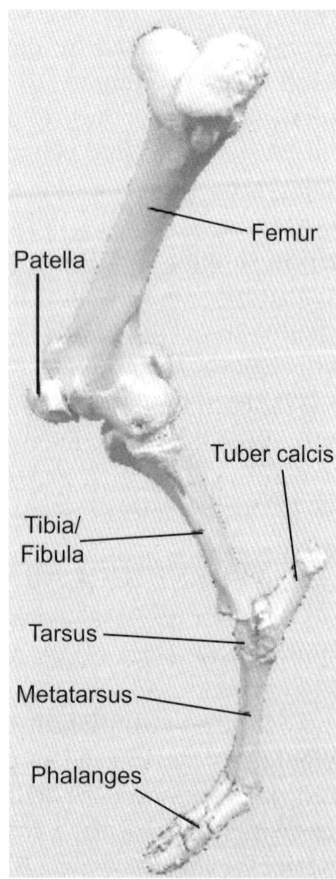

HINDLEG

As with the foreleg, the hind leg can be considered to be anomalous with the human leg. The large femur articulates proximally with the acetabulum of the pelvis in a ball and socket synovial joint, it is further secured in this joint by the presence of a round ligament (*lig. capitis*). The femur articulates distally with the tibia and rudimentary fibula at the stifle joint. Cranial to this joint, articulating with the femur is the patella (kneecap), held in position by three ligaments which also connect the patella to the tibia and fibula the latter of which is rudimentary and partially fused to the tibia, but is important as the distal end forms part of the hock joint.

The tibia articulates with two rows of tarsal bones, two in the upper row, three in the lower, the arrangement of which allows for flexion and extension of the hock. The rear of the hock is formed by the *Tuber calcis* situated at the rear of the top row which represents the point of attachment of the biceps and gastrocnemius muscles. The metatarsus is longer than the corresponding metacarpus of the forelimb and articulates distally with the two digits each formed by three phalanges.

ANATOMY OF THE FOOT

The hooves support the entire weight of the animal and can also be diagnostic of certain disease and welfare conditions in addition to being an obvious entry portal to inoculated pathogens present in the environment.

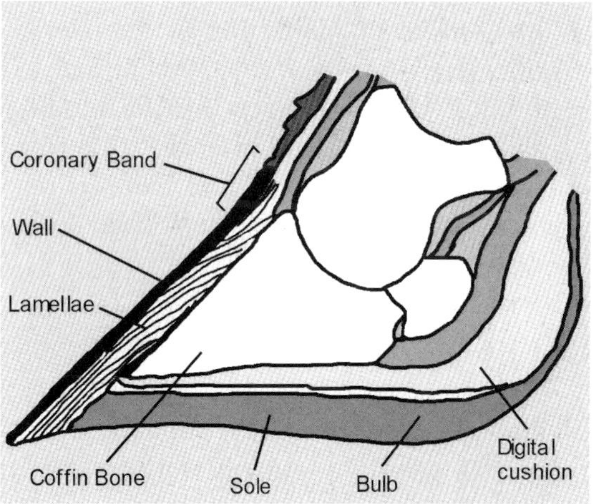

The heel of the hoof is formed by the bulb and digital cushion, the former being composed of soft rubbery horn material and the internal digital cushion acting as an elastic shock absorber.

Attached to the coffin bone, the terminal phalange, are laminae, formed by horn growth. In normal situations wear of the wall and laminae is equal to their growth, however cattle kept on soft ground will frequently display extended growth of the horn which eventually leads to lameness as stress is placed on parts of the hoof not intended to be in contact with the ground.

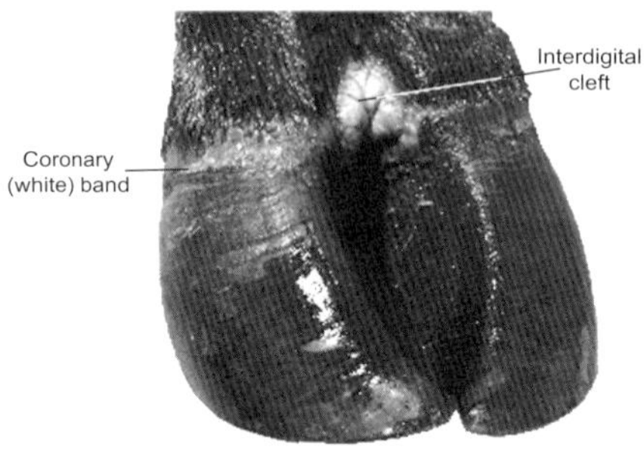

Front of hoof

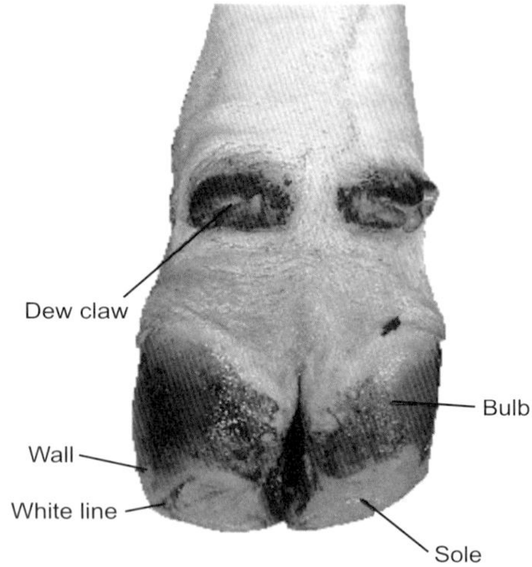

Rear of hoof

MUSCLE

INTRODUCTION

Muscle is the reason that the meat animals are reared and slaughtered; the post mortem changes that occur in muscle converting it to meat. In the live animal muscle is found anchored to the skeletal frame providing posture, an ability to move and protection for the internal organs. It also appears internally to provide movement in the viscera and to provide valves to regulate flow, achieving this by converting the chemical energy of ATP (Adenosine triphosphate) to mechanical energy. There are three types of muscle; Skeletal muscle, cardiac muscle, and smooth muscle, each possessing different characteristics. Cardiac muscle will be dealt with in the cardiovascular system later.

SKELETAL MUSCLE

This is also known as striated muscle and is under semi voluntary control of the nervous system and generally contracts around a fulcrum to facilitate movement about a joint.

ANATOMY OF MUSCLE

Muscle is composed of individual long muscle fibres enclosed by a collagenous membrane, the endomysium, grouped into bundles surrounded by a second membrane called the perimysium. These bundles are further enclosed by the epimysium to form the muscle proper. The epimysium membrane extends past the termination of the muscle fibres to form the tendons that attach the muscles to the bone via the periosteum.

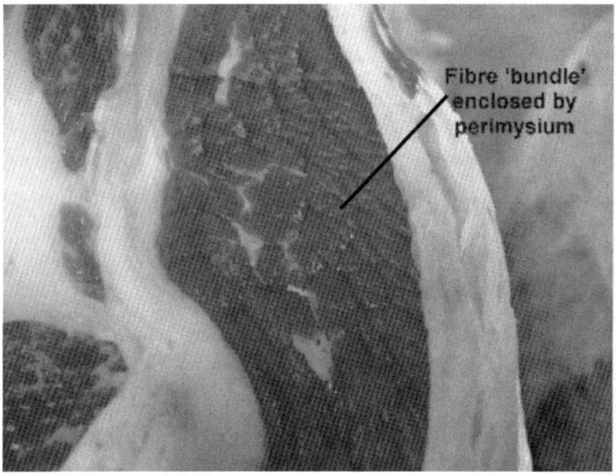

FIBRES

Fibres are formed by the fusion of muscle cells (myoblasts) and hence each fibre contains numerous nuclei and mitochondria. Each fibre contains filaments of protein, the interaction of which in the presence of ATP coverts chemical energy into mechanical energy. Thick filaments are formed by the protein myosin, a protein that contains areas that have an affinity for bonding with ATP and also the protein forming the thinner filaments actin.

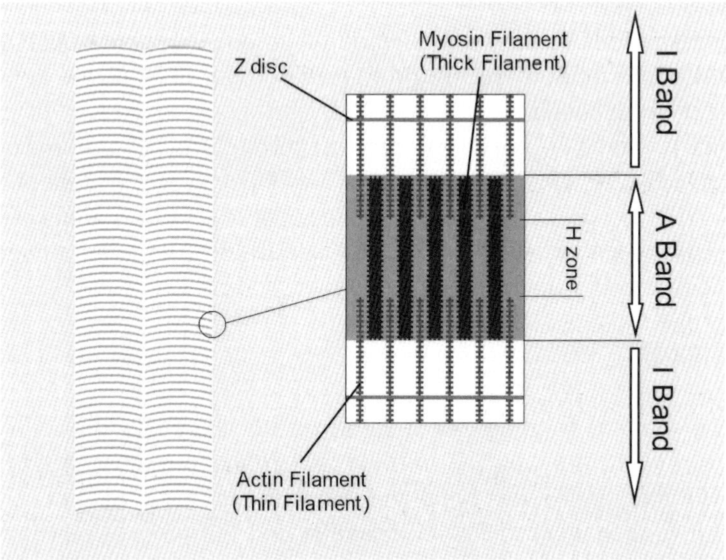

The term striated muscle is given as, microscopically, bands are visible within the muscle fibre which corresponds to the degree of overlap of these protein filaments in a given area.

The banding noted in the muscle is given nomenclature, the dark bands are due to the thick filaments of myosin and are termed the A-band, and conversely the I-band is due to the presence of the thinner actin filaments. The area where the two types of filaments do not overlap is called the H-zone. The I-band is bisected by the Z-disc which is a band of non-contractile protein to which the myofibrils are attached; the area between two Z-discs forms the sarcolemma, the functional contractile unit of muscle.

ATP- ADENOSINE TRIPHOSPHATE

ATP is a compound formed by the hydrolysis of nucleic acids known as a nucleotide. It exists in all cells of the body and provides the main energy storage unit, a type of battery that stores energy in the form of high-energy phosphate bonds on the molecule. During muscular contraction the ATP molecule breaks the bond between the actin and myosin filaments but loses a phosphate group in the process releasing energy. The ATP now converts to adenosine diphosphate (ADP).

A small amount of ATP is stored in muscle cells; once this has been exhausted the muscle fibre will fatigue as the lactic acid level raises and will cease to function. The replacement of ATP is achieved in three ways, each method producing a phosphate bond to convert ADP to ATP; cellular respiration, conversion of creatine phosphate and conversion of glycogen. When these methods are exhausted the myosin/actin bonds become permanent.

Cellular respiration is the main method of producing enough ATP to meet the demands of the muscle during prolonged activity and for the conversion of lactic acid to glycogen.

Glycogen is stored in muscle fibres and through the glycolytic pathway reaction converts ADP to ATP by breakdown of lactic acid. Creatine phosphate reacts with ADP to produce ATP and creatine. These latter reactions are finite; once they have been exhausted cellular respiration provides the energy for ATP production in the muscle.

CONTRACTION

On receiving stimulus from the nerve the myosin head attracts the actin toward it and binds with it, drawing the unfixed thin filament along the fixed thick filament. ATP then breaks this bond and the actin rebinds at the next available myosin head further down the thick filament and the process repeats having the effect of shortening the sarcomere in a gear toothed or ratchet-like manner. During contraction the A-band (the darker band) remains the same size, the I-band shortens as the Z-discs are pulled toward each other.

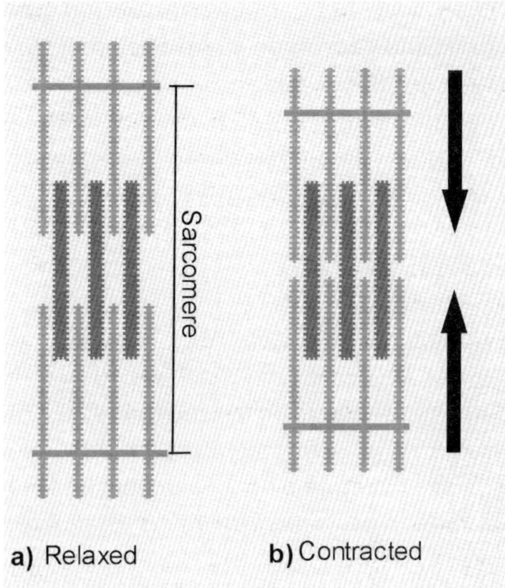

FIBRE TYPES

Two types of fibre are found in a muscle group, Type I (red fibres) and Type II (white fibres) that have different characteristics as listed below. The combination of these fibres within a muscle determines that muscles efficiency for the tasks required of it.

Type I Fibre	Type II Fibre
Red fibre (Slow Twitch)	White Fibre (Fast Twitch)
Large number of mitochondria	Low number of mitochondria
Dependent on cellular respiration ATP	Dependent on Glycolytic ATP
Rich in myoglobin	Low in myoglobin
Activated by small diameter (slow conducting) neurons	Activated by large diameter (fast conducting) neurons
Fatigue resistant	Used for rapid contraction
More prevalent in muscles of posture	Fatigue easily
	More dominant in muscles used for rapid movement.

RIGOR MORTIS

Rigor mortis, the 'death stiffening' that occurs after death is the permanent bonding of the myosin/actin filaments once the available ATP is exhausted due to the lack of cellular respiration. The process of rigor mortis has three phases: A **delay phase** during which time available ATP is used within the muscle fibre to prevent myosin/actin bonding. An **onset phase** during which time the cellular respiration ATP is exhausted and the pool of ATP from creatine phosphate and glycolysis are used up and permanent rigor myosin/actin bonds are formed, and a final **completion phase** where the regeneration of ATP ceases and the myosin/actin filaments become fully bonded. These bonds eventually break due to the lower pH conditions that occur in the carcase. It is worth mentioning that the hardening of fat is not due to rigor but to the lowering of temperature.

NERVE SUPPLY

Each individual muscle fibre is served by an axon that branches from a motor neuron (see nerves types and function in Nervous System section). Stimulation of the motor neuron creates contraction within every fibre served by the braches of its axon, therefore muscles requiring precise control will be served by many neurons with few branches, and large muscles can be controlled by few motor neurons with many branches

SMOOTH MUSCLE

Smooth muscle, also known as visceral muscle is found within the walls of the hollow structures of the body with the notable exception of the heart. Contraction of smooth muscle alters the dimension of the structures including the diameter of arteries, the peristaltic motion of the intestines, the diameter of the bronchi, contraction of the urinary bladder during urination, and contraction of the uterus during parturition.

Unlike cardiac and skeletal muscle there are no visible strata within smooth muscle, although it still contains the sliding filaments of actin and myosin but fixed to the cell membrane rather than a Z-disc. Smooth muscle comprises single cells that posses contractile properties. The contraction of smooth muscle is partially involuntary as is cardiac muscle, but can also be stimulated by motor neurons and the presence of hormones. For example the presence of bile in the small intestine has a triggering effect on the peristaltic movement of the intestinal smooth muscle, and oxytocin released into the bloodstream stimulates contraction of the uterus at parturition.

THE RESPIRATORY SYSTEM

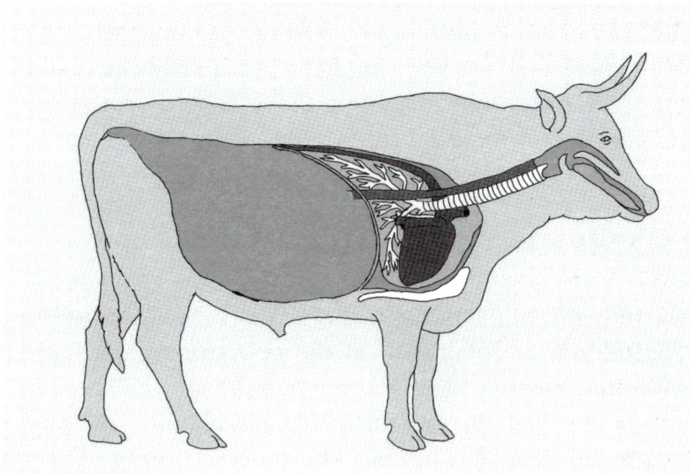

INTRODUCTION

The tissue cells of the body require oxygen to function; they also require the removal of the waste products of their metabolism, including carbon dioxide. The cardiovascular system is the transport vector by which this is achieved, the respiratory system being the method of gaseous exchange of oxygen for carbon dioxide, voiding the latter from the body. For the purposes of description the respiratory system will be considered as the nostrils, nasal passages, larynx, trachea, bronchi and the lungs.

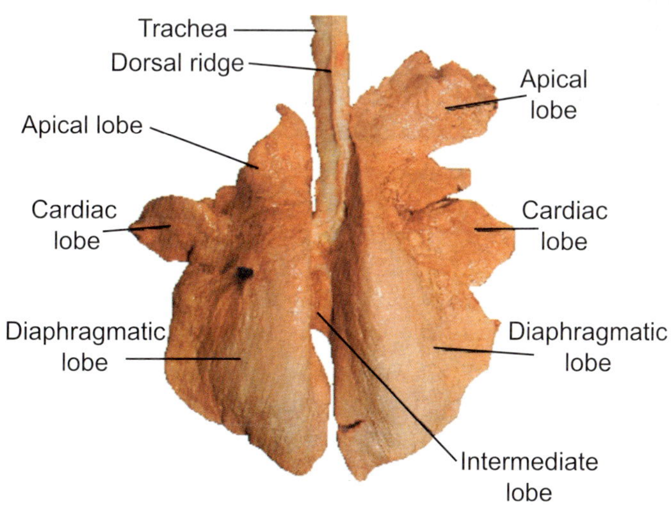

Bovine lungs

DISTINCTIVE FEATURES

The bovine trachea is long, made up of 50+ cartilaginous rings and possesses a dorsal ridge. There are two main bronchi and a single accessory bronchus leading to the right apical lobe. The lung tissue is soft, spongy and lobulated. The left lung consists of three lobes; the right consists of four or five lobes.

NOSTRILS AND NASAL PASSAGES

Air is drawn into the body through the nostrils, the size of which can be varied by contraction or relaxation of the surrounding cartilage reinforced muscles. Inside the nostrils begins a mucous lining which covers the scroll like turbinate bones that lie ventral to the nasal bone, the shape of these bones forces the inspired air against the mucous lining. The presence of mucous on hairs inside the nostrils serves as a trap for foreign particulate matter above 10μm in diameter, and also, in conjunction with the heavily vascularised nasal tissue, serves to moisten and warm the inspired air before it continues to the larynx.

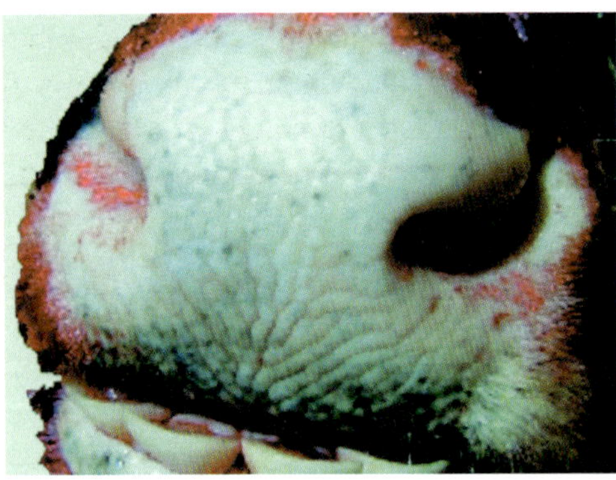

Bovine muzzle

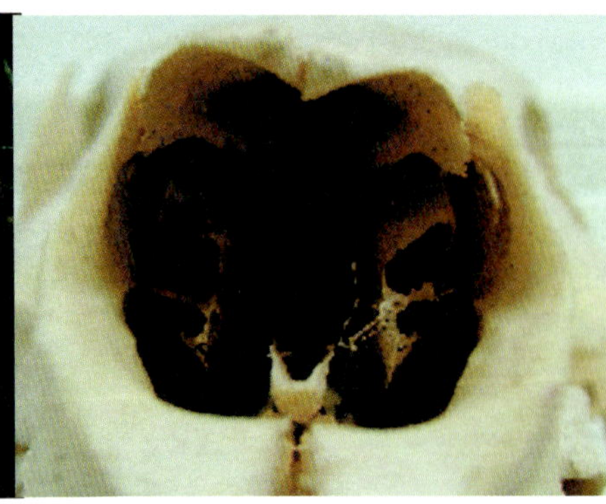

Turbinate bones

LARYNX

The larynx is formed from five cartilaginous structures that articulate with each other. The main body of the larynx is formed by the cricoid and thyroid cartilages. Within this body are two arytenoid cartilages that articulate with the thyroid cartilage and form the mechanism of vocalisation of the animal. Cranial to the paired arytenoids cartilages is the epiglottis, which also articulates with the thyroid cartilage, this structure moves to cover the opening of the larynx during swallowing to prevent the aspiration of foodstuffs into the trachea.

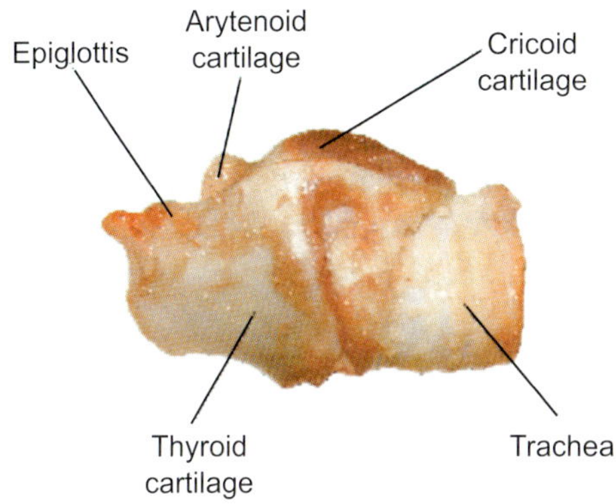

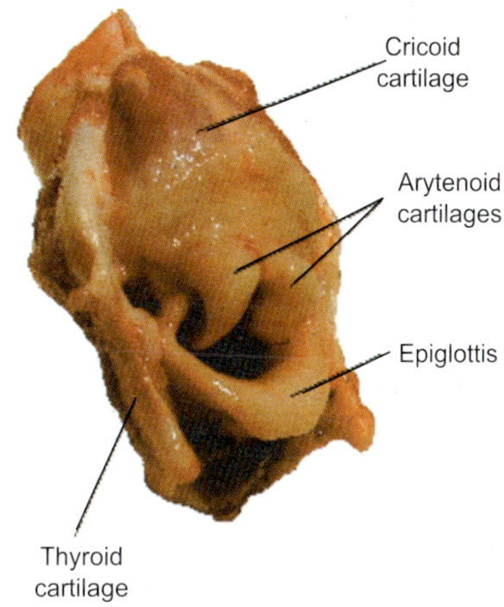

TRACHEA

The trachea (windpipe) is given structure by approximately 50 cartilaginous incomplete rings that prevent the collapse of this tube during the low pressure encountered during respiration. These incomplete rings meet behind the trachea forming a prominent dorsal ridge that can be used as an aid when identifying specimens. The internal structure of the trachea includes ciliated cells and mucosal cells forming part of the bodies' immune response, catching particles larger than 2µm and removing them by the escalatory peristaltic motion of the cilia to the larynx and pharynx where expectoration expels them from the body.

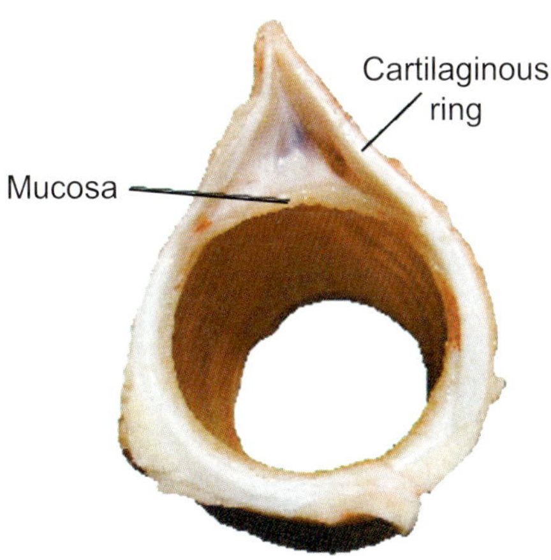

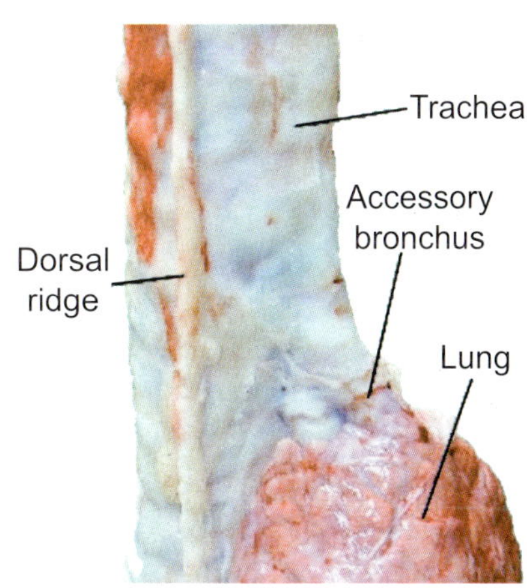

BRONCHI

The trachea branches off into the smaller diameter bronchi on entrance to the lung tissue. In cattle a cranial accessory bronchus branches off the trachea to the right apical lobe before the two main bronchi divide the trachea at the point known as the bifurcation. The bronchi then further subdivide within the lung tissue forming the air passageway known as the bronchial tree the branches of which continue to subdivide until they reach microscopic terminal sacs, the alveoli also known as air sacs.

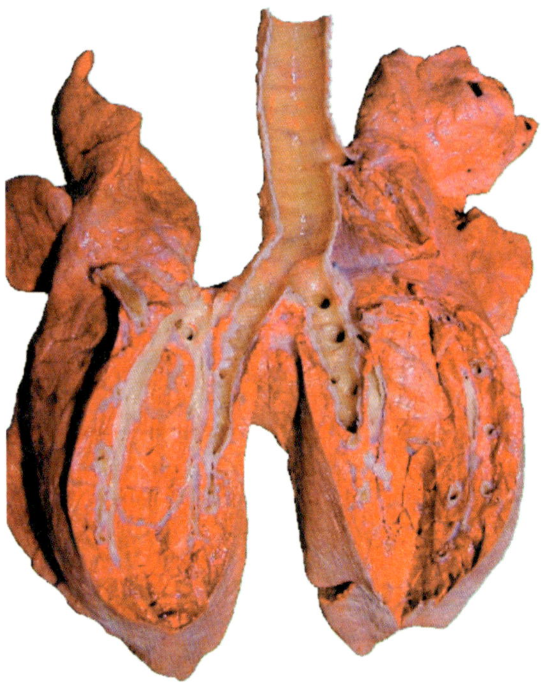

Dissection of the trachea and bronchi of bovine lungs

The alveoli, which are surrounded by a web of interjoining capillaries, are formed by alveolar cells attached to a thin gas permeable basement membrane which separates them from the capillaries. The alveolar cells are constantly dividing and have the ability to move from their position to undertake their role as part of the bodies' immune system. The alveolar cells have phagocytic properties, and can absorb particles less than 2μm in diameter and remove them by entering lymphatic vessels in the surrounding tissue.

THE ACT OF RESPIRATION

During inspiration the muscles of the diaphragm contract pulling it flat and tight. This, combined with the simultaneous contraction of the intercostal muscles that increases the diameter of the thorax, creates a reduction in the internal air pressure which leads to atmospheric air being drawn in to equalize the pressure. Exhalation involves a relaxation of the muscles that increases the internal pressure and air is drawn out of the body in another attempt to equalize pressure.

The air is drawn through the nostrils, down the trachea and to the alveoli via the bronchial tree where it diffuses through the alveolal wall into the blood. Haemoglobin in the erythrocytes binds oxygen in this circumstance, where the partial oxygen pressure is high, and releases carbon dioxide which moves into the alveoli for expulsion. The oxygen is then carried to the tissue cells of the body where the reduced partial oxygen pressure causes disassociation and release of the oxygen converting the oxyhaemoglobin back to haemoglobin in which state, in conjunction with the reduced partial oxygen pressure, carbon dioxide is absorbed.

DIGESTIVE SYSTEM

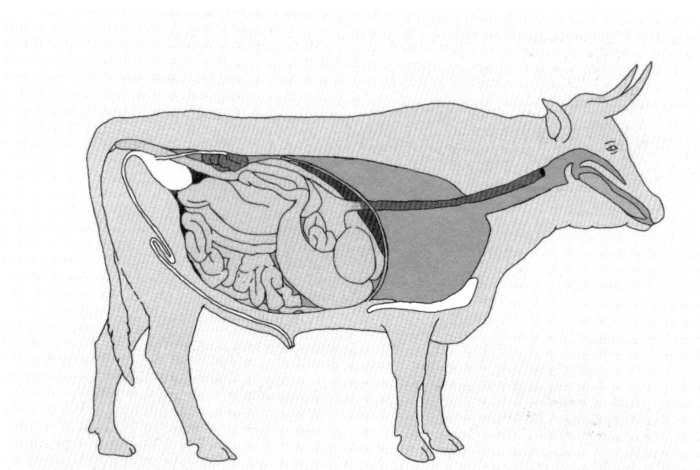

INTRODUCTION

The purpose of the digestive system is the conversion of in- taken fuel (food) into basic components that are either water-soluble or to particles small enough to be held in suspension in solution. In this form these components can be removed from the digestive system, and transported through the body for synthesis into complex chemicals, storage etc. The digestive system achieves this conversion by means of mechanical and biochemical mechanisms aided by the length of the intestines and immense surface area available for absorption of these nutrients which are then transported through the body by both the blood circulation and the lymphatic system. The digestive system can be considered as a tube of varying diameter stretching from the mouth to the anus.

THE MOUTH

The mouth, or buccal cavity, provides the initial stages of digestion, mechanical and chemical. The upper hard palate, the mandible, the soft tissue pharynx at the rear, and the lips at the front, form this cavity. The sides of the buccal cavity are formed by the cheeks, the purpose of which is to expand to allow more food into the cavity but possess enough elastic capability to move food back into the central cavity for further processing by chewing (mastication). The inner surfaces of the cheeks of cattle are protected from penetrative damage by hard or sharp items of herbage by conical buccal papillae.

There are three pairs of salivary glands secreting a fluid containing mucin to moisten the food as it is chewed and reduce froth in the rumen, a cause of bloat. In addition saliva contains sodium and potassium bicarbonate to buffer the acidity of the rumen, and mineral salts to aid bacterial growth. These are situated at the rear of the mouth near the base of the jaw (submaxillary), in front of the insertion of the ear (parotid) and in a sub mucosal layer lateral to the tongue (sublingual).

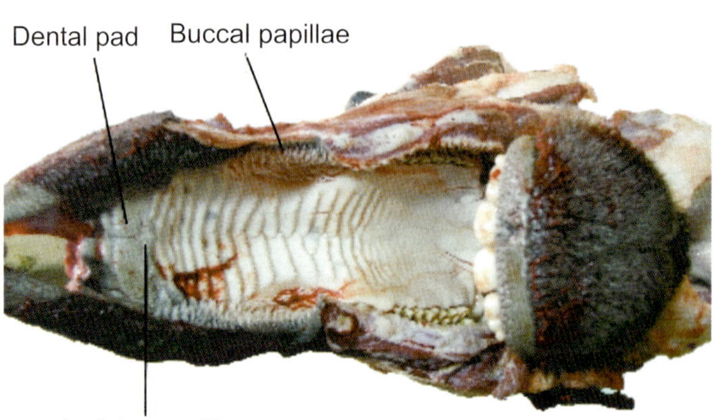

The bovine upper palate possesses no incisors, food being sheared by the action of the lower incisors against the hard, keratinised dental pad. The hard upper palate extends dorsally joining the soft palate that in turn joins the pharynx. The soft palate is bordered by the upper molars that move in a grinding action against those of the lower jaw.

Movement of the mandible is mainly achieved through contraction of the external masseter muscles and the internal pterygoid muscles. At the front of the mandible are the incisors. Initial temporary (deciduous) incisors are replaced by permanent counterparts over time, the eruption of this permanent dentition being, (given the vagaries of genetics and chance), both systematic and predictable and therefore used as a method of approximating the age of cattle.

ESTIMATION OF AGE USING DENTITION

0 permanent incisors.
Birth –2 weeks

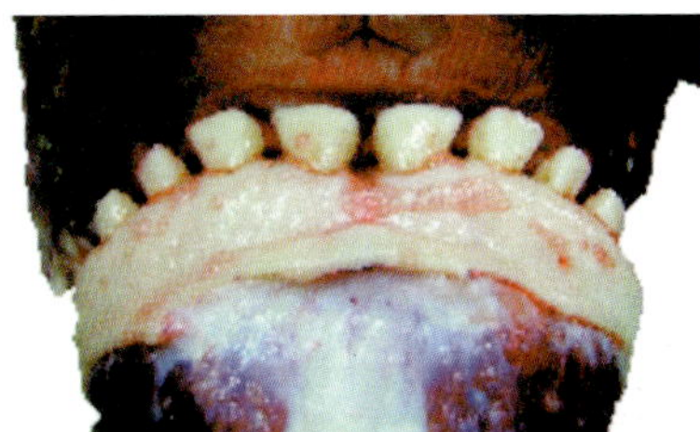

2 permanent incisors.
18-24 months

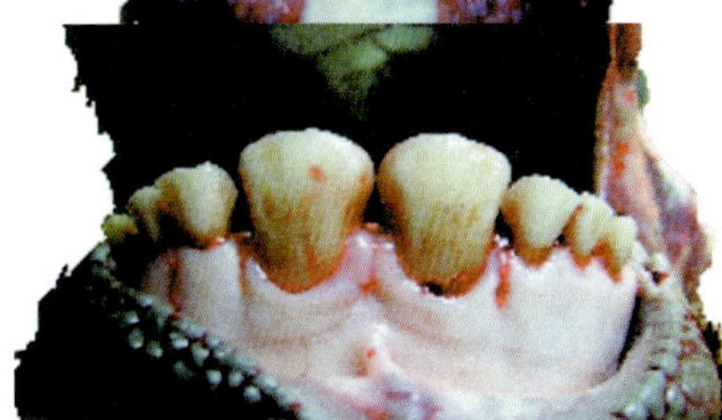

4 permanent incisors.
24-30 months

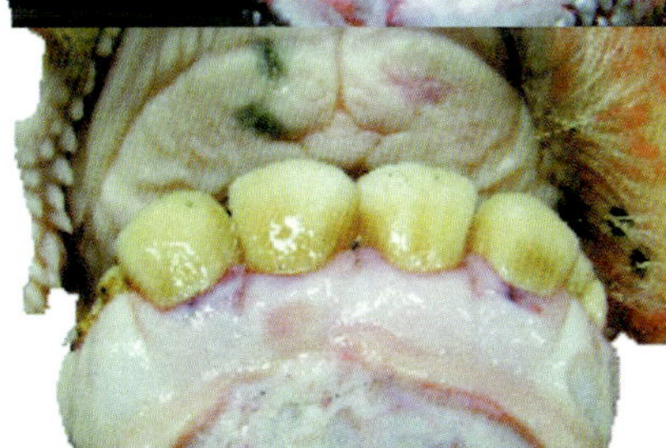

6 permanent incisors.
36-42 months

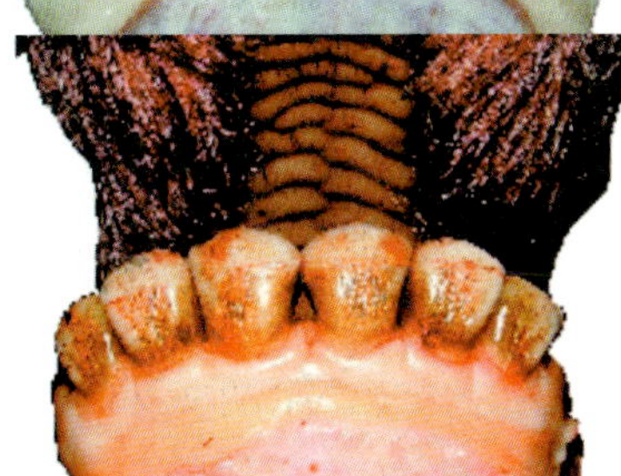

THE TONGUE

This is a muscular, occasionally pigmented, semi- prehensile organ used to draw food into the buccal cavity where it is severed by the action of the incisors against the upper dental pad. The shape of the tongue conforms to the basic shape of the lower jaw and it is rooted at the base to the hyoid bone at the rear of the mandible.

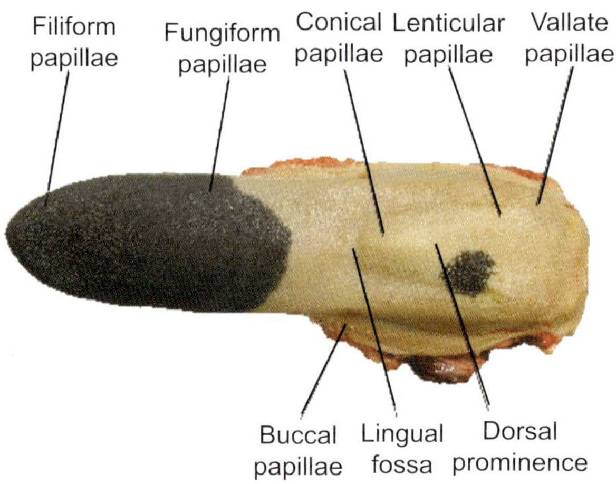

The dorsal surface of the tongue is distinguished by the presence of various characteristic lingual papillae. The tip of the tongue is roughened by horny, rearward facing filiform (threadlike) papillae, scattered amongst these are fungiform (mushroom like) papillae. Approximately half way along the dorsal surface of the tongue is a transverse depression in front of a dorsal prominence, the latter being covered in lenticular (lens like) papillae. Toward the rear of this prominence, either side of the midline a group of 7-10 vallate (rim like), papillae, which in conjunction with the fungiform papillae constitute the taste buds.

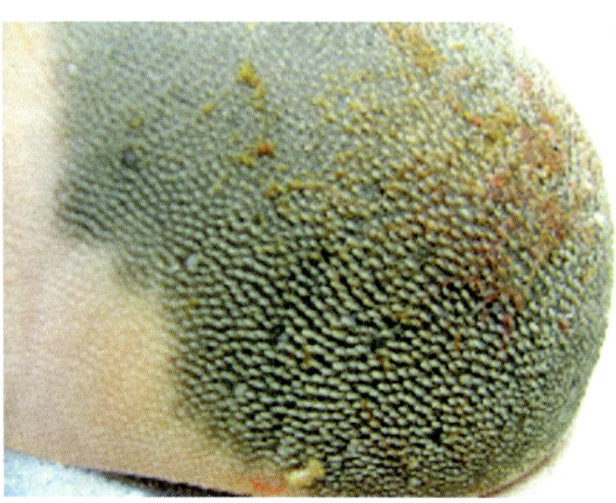

Filiform papillae

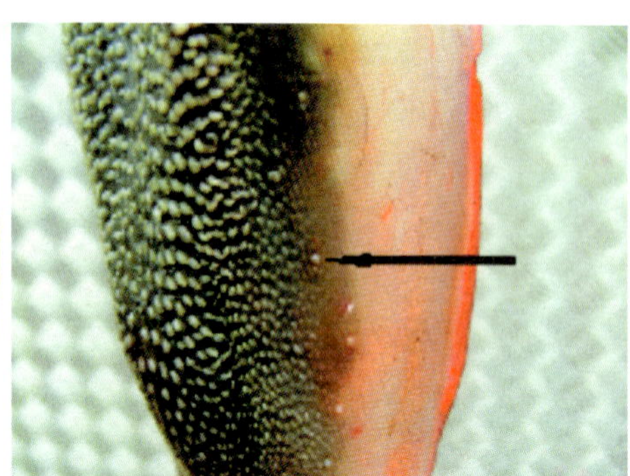

Fungiform papillae (arrowed)

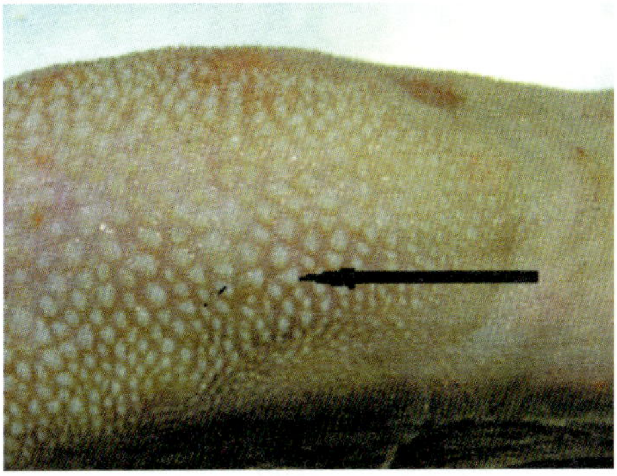

Lenticular papillae (arrowed)

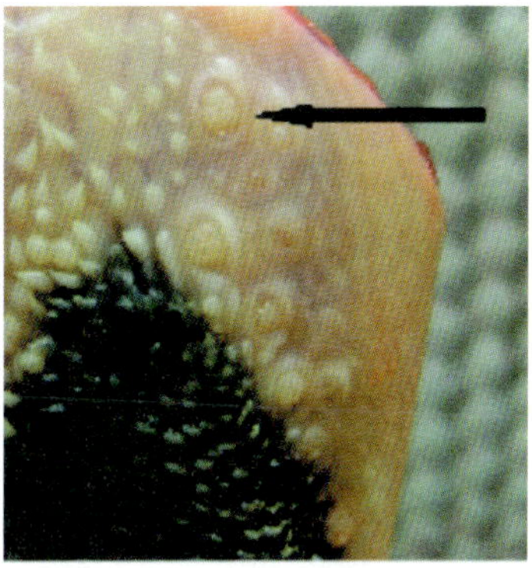

Vallate papillae (arrowed)

OESOPHAGUS

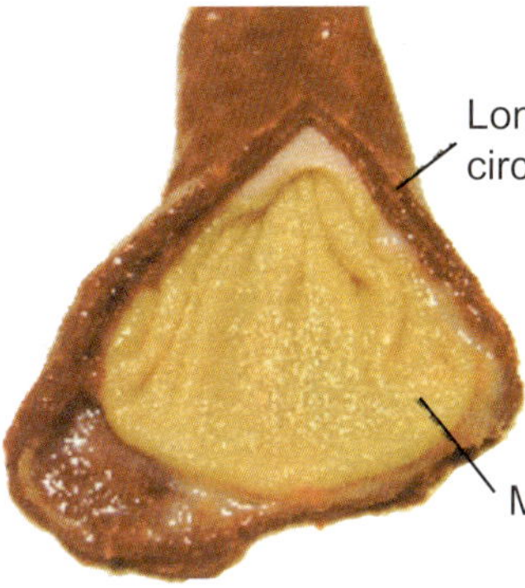

This runs from the pharynx to the rumen, the fore stomach. The oesophagus is a mucosal lined tube, surrounded by an inner layer of circular muscle encapsulated in a sheath of longitudinal muscle. When these muscles contract they produce a wave like motion (peristalysis) squeezing food material down the length of the oesophagus. In ruminant animals such as cattle, this action is partly under conscious control, allowing material to be moved back up the oesophagus from the fore stomach to the mouth for further mastication.

FORESTOMACHS

In the ruminant animal, the digestion of rough complex carbohydrates requires a degree of fermentation to occur by bacterial action. This is accomplished in the forestomachs, comprising the three chambers of the rumen, reticulum and omasum. The abomasum being the true or gastric stomach. The walls of the forestomachs comprise a smooth peritoneal covering, a thick muscular layer (involuntary muscle arranged in circular, oblique and longitudinal layers to provide a churning of the contents), a submucosal layer of connective tissue and a thick mucous membrane.

RUMEN

This chamber communicates directly with the reticulum. An internal groove (reticular or oesophageal groove) directs food from the oesophagus into both chambers. The rumen occupies a large percentage of the abdominal cavity mostly on the left hand side, accounting for approximately 80% of the volume of the stomachs. The interior mucosa of the rumen is covered with keratinised papillae that range from a leaf form to barely visible conical papillae at the roof of the rumen.

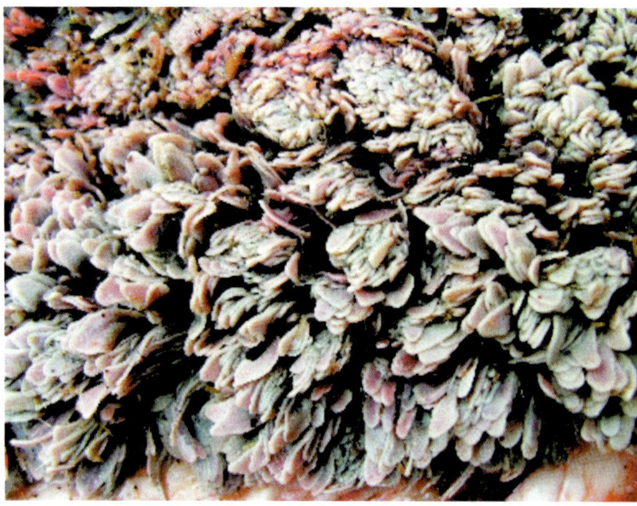

Detail of the leaf-like papillae of the rumen

The contents of the rumen tend to form layers, the lower layers being made up of remasticated fermenting material, the upper layers of less dense material awaiting regurgitation up the oesophagus for further chewing, with a final layer of gas. The capacity of the rumen ranges from 120-200 litres of ingested feed and water in the adult.

RETICULUM

Also known as the honeycomb due to the shape of the areas of the mucosa that are enclosed by ridges. The reticulum is situated cranial to the rumen and receives a percentage of the oesophageal discharge, generally the remasticated denser material. It is thought that a portion of the volatile fatty acids produced during the bacterial fermentation of the complex carbohydrates are absorbed through the mucosa of the rumen and reticulum and that the structure of the internal mucosa of the reticulum provides an increased surface area for this to occur.

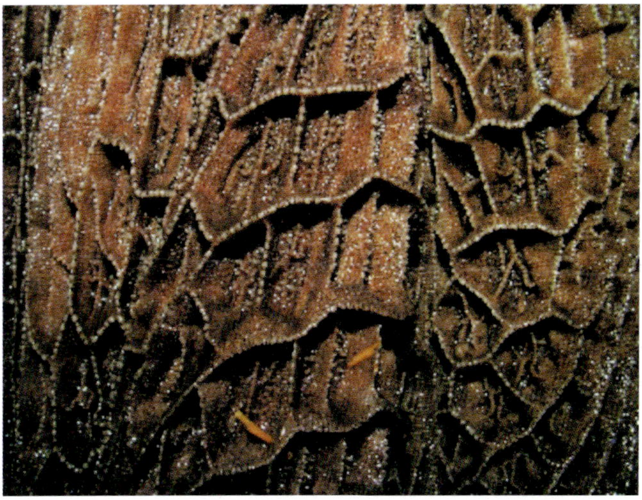

Rumen detail of internal wall

The uneven surface of the reticulum also allows penetration of sharp or hard objects through the mucosal wall, which combined with the anatomical position of the reticulum against the diaphragm and in relation to the heart can lead to a traumatic pericarditis or peritonitis, known as 'hardware disease'.

OMASUM

The omasum, colloquially known as 'manyplies' or 'bible' is the third and smallest and final forestomach of bovines. Internally the mucosal surface is heavily folded into laminae hence the synonyms, these laminae being covered in lenticular and conical papillae. Ingesta enters via the reticulo-omasal orifice and exits into the abomasum through an omasal-abomasal orifice. Contractions of the omasum force ingesta between the laminae and further into the abomasum.

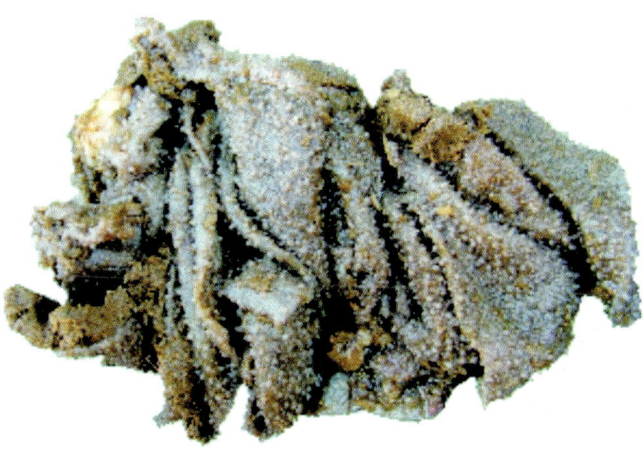

A portion of omasum, demonstrating laminae and lenticular papillae.

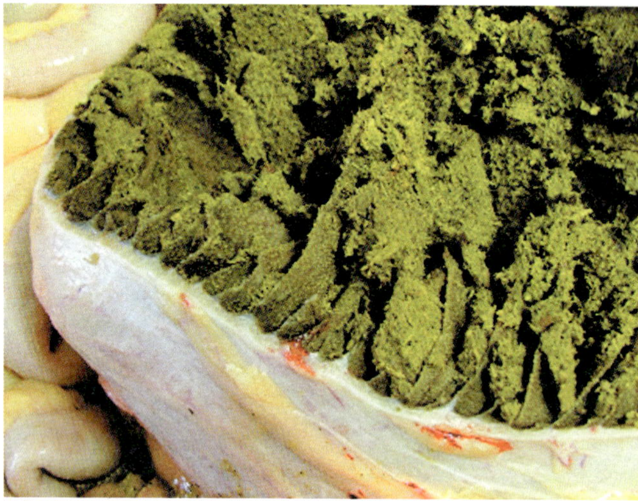

Incision into an omasum, demonstrating laminae and ingesta

ABOMASUM

The abomasum represents the true gastric stomach of the ruminant animal. Once fermented the ingesta passes from the omasum into the abomasum, the internal mucosal surface of which is generally pink and glandular as opposed to the greenish discolouration of the previous forestomachs.

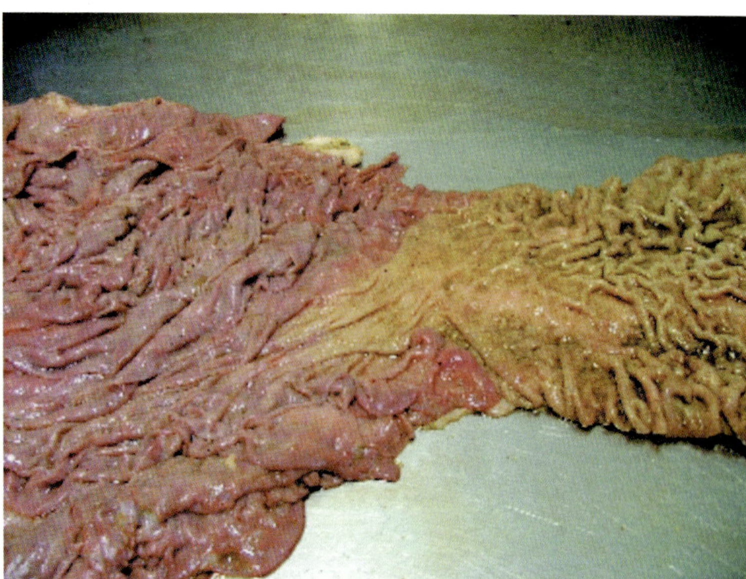

Opened and cleaned abomasum

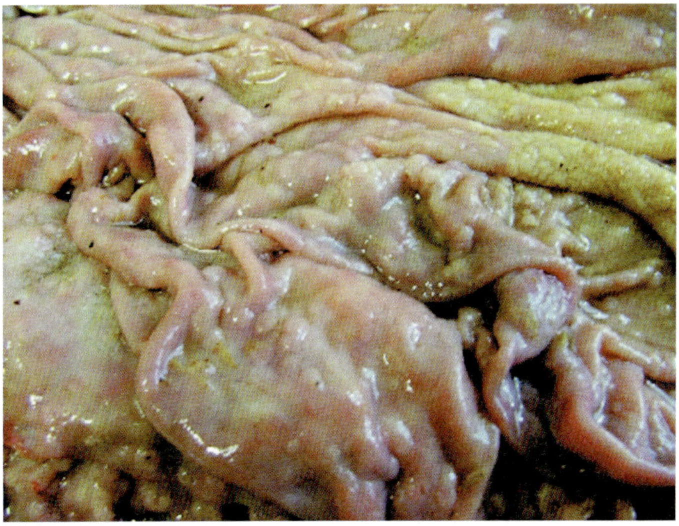

Detail of the gastric glands of the abomasal mucosa

RUMINATION

Once the in taken food has undergone the initial process of mastication and mixing with saliva it is swallowed, moves down the oesophagus by peristaltic motion and enters the rumen. Here the ingesta are subjected to the churning motion of the stomach and the presence of cellulose splitting bacteria aided by the alkalinity of the saliva. After a period of time in the rumen a bolus of the ingesta is regurgitated by contraction of the rumen and reverse peristalsis of the oesophagus back to the mouth where it is re-chewed with the addition of more saliva to begin the process of converting starches to sugars. The food is then re-swallowed.

The rumen contains bacteria and protozoa that produce surface enzymes to break down food and synthesise the by-products of fermentation such as volatile fatty acids (VFAs) and vitamins B and K, the VFAs being absorbed directly through the rumen. The gaseous by products of the fermentation process, carbon dioxide and methane are mostly voided from the rumen by eructation (belching).

Which compartment of the stomach the ingesta then enters is dependant on its state of maceration and specific gravity, if still requiring fermentation and maceration it is heavy and re-enters the rumen, if highly fluid and well macerated it passes into the omasum. The omasum has the sole function of grinding the ingesta into a paste before it enters the abomasum. The food is forced through the leaves of the omasum and is subjected to grinding by the keratinised papillae and the muscular action of the omasal walls. Finally the food paste enters the abomasum. Throughout the passage and storage of the ingesta in the forestomachs, cellulose- splitting bacteria break down the fibres of the herbage.

The glands in the mucous membrane of the abomasum secretes gastric juice which contains enzymes such as pepsin and rennin in addition to hydrochloric acid. In this acidic environment fat and peptones are released, lysozyme enzyme is also released which breaks down bacterial cell walls destroying bacteria before they enter the small intestines The food then enters the intestines via the pyloric sphincter.

THE INTESTINES

The intestines are generally divided into the small intestine consisting of the duodenum, jejunum and ileum, and the large intestines of the caecum, colon and rectum.

SMALL INTESTINE

The small intestine runs from the pyloric sphincter of the abomasum to the ileo-caecal valve. Although the small intestines do secrete a nominal amount of enzymes, their primary function is the absorption of released nutrients. The walls of the intestines are formed, anomalous with the forestomachs by four layers; a thin peritoneal surface, two muscular layers, longitudinal and lateral, and an inner mucosal layer. In addition to mucosal folds (rugae) the internal mucosa of the intestines is lined with microvilli, finger-like projections into the lumen that greatly increase the surface area of the intestines but also act as the main points through which nutrients are absorbed. The villi encapsulate a central lymph channel surrounded by blood capillaries. Situated in the mucosa and submucosa are raised patches of lymphoid follicles collectively known as Peyer's patches (see Lymphatic system).

Duodenum

The duodenum is divided into two ascending and a single descending portion. The ascending portion starts at the pyloric sphincter and follows a vertical path to the visceral surface of the liver to which it is attached by a portion of the omentum (a fold of the peritoneum), followed by a descending portion running toward the pelvic region before ascending again to a point of attachment with the mesentery, (a further membranous peritoneal fold attaching organs to the abdominal wall). The pancreatic duct joins the descending duodenum, and the bile duct enters at a point where the duodenum is held to the visceral hepatic surface.

Jejunum

The jejunum continues from the point at which the duodenum enters the periphery of the mesentery and follows the extremities of this to join the ileum. The jejunum is shadowed by a parallel line of mesenteric lymph nodes situated further within the substance of the mesentery, embedded in fat.

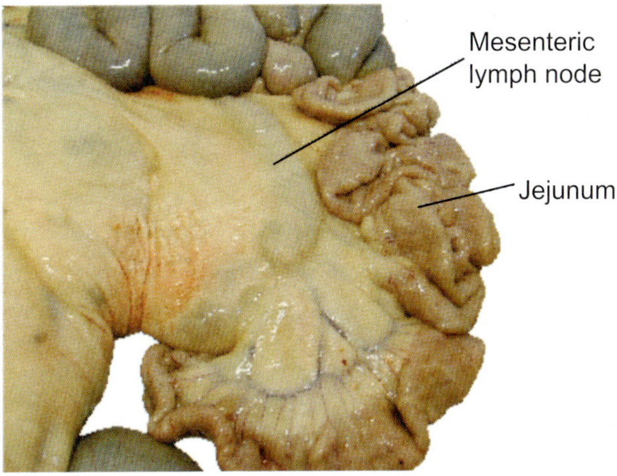

Ileum

The ileum is short and terminates at the ileo-caecal valve.

LARGE INTESTINE

The large intestine is mainly involved in water balance and the absorption of minerals and volatile fatty acids. The caecum also acts as a secondary fermentation vessel, bacterial activity providing further break down of the food. The large intestine primarily secretes mucous to aid movement of material and terminates at the rectum, or anus, where the waste matter is voided from the body.

Caecum

Starting at the ileo caecal valve (a valve that performs a similar function to the pyloric sphincter, preventing the contents of the caecum from extruding back into the ileum during muscular contraction) the caecum is a blind ended diverticula of the large intestine. The end of the caecum is loosely attached allowing vertical movement of the sac dependant on the volume of gas it contains.

Colon

The colon is of a similar diameter to the undistended caecum and is positioned within the mesentery where it narrows in diameter and follows a winding clockwise diminishing spiral pattern for 1½-2 turns before returning in an anticlockwise spiral to join the free transverse section of colon that leads to the rectum. The main function of the colon is maintenance of the water balance, the removal of water from the faecal matter before entering the rectum. The mucosa of the colon secretes mucous to lubricate the faecal matter.

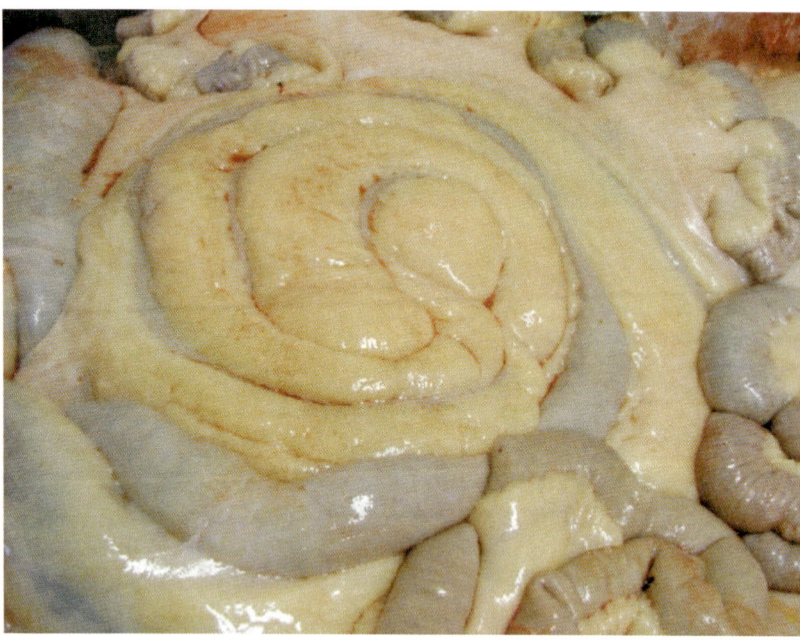

The spiral of the colon, embedded in mesenteric fat

Rectum

This area stores faecal matter prior to expulsion through the anus. The rectum has a larger calibre than the colon with muscular walls. This leads to the anus which comprises an orifice controlled by an internal and external sphincter, the latter of which is comprised of skeletal muscle and hence is under conscious control.

INTESTINAL FUNCTION AND DIGESTION

After the foodstuff has undergone initial enzyme degradation and been subjected to the acid conditions of the abomasum (pH>2) the resultant fluid paste enters the duodenum through the pyloric sphincter. This involuntary muscle prevents the reflux of the ingesta back to the abomasum. The muscular layers of the intestinal wall then move the food by peristaltic motion, this propels the food through the intestine, has a 'mixing' affect and also forces the food against the absorptive lining of the mucosa.

The bile received in the cranial duodenum stimulates peristaltic contraction of the intestinal muscles, and in conjunction with the pancreatic juice reduces fats to free fatty acids and emulsifies them to enable their removal through the lymphatic channels of the villi. This fat removal generally takes place in the jejunum giving the lymph channels leading from the intestines a milky appearance known as 'chyle'. This fluid collects in the *Cisterna chyli* and then enters the blood circulation at the thoracic duct.

In the presence of pancreatic enzymes, proteins are degraded to amino acids and peptides, starches are reduced to glucose and other sugars and absorbed directly into the capillary beds surrounding the villi and thence to the liver via the hepatic portal vein.

THE LIVER

APPEARANCE

The bovine liver is a dark brown colour, with a smooth convex outer surface and consists of three lobes, a left and right lobe indistinctly separated at an umbilical fissure, a caudate lobe, and a rounded gall bladder partially imbedded in the liver substance. The liver possesses several depressions where it is in contact with other organs. The left lobe is thinner than the right, bearing the impression of the reticulum against which it rests in the live animal. This lobe is bordered by the umbilical fissure (which occasionally bears a remnant of the umbilicus) and the oesophageal notch. The thicker right lobe is compressed by the presence of the omasum. At the centre of this lobe, normally covered by the pancreas is situated the entry point of the portal vein and artery into the liver surrounded by the hepatic lymph nodes, and also indicates the point at which the cystic duct leaves the liver for the gall bladder.

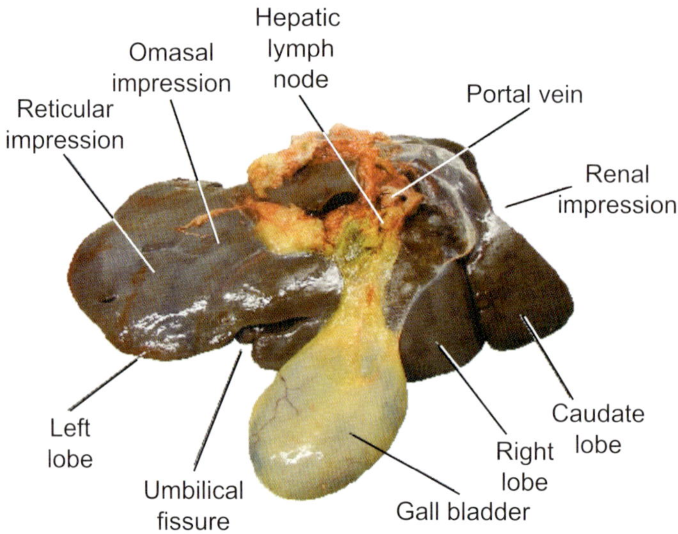

Bovine liver – Visceral surface

Joined to the right lobe of the liver is the square ended caudate lobe which blends with the right lobe at a depression formed by the presence of the right kidney, the renal impression.

When the liver is removed from the carcase a segment of the posterior vena cava remains attached.

LIVER STRUCTURE

The liver is mainly composed of small filtration and secretion units called lobules. Each lobule is enclosed in a thin connective tissue and comprises specialist liver cells, including the main liver cells, hepatocytes, surrounding a central capillary of the hepatic portal vein. The hepatocytes are segregated from the blood vessels by a basement membrane covered with basic epithelial cells and the phagocytic Kupfer cells. The hepatocytes are closely packed together but do have small canals between them that collect the produced bile and then connect together to form a network that eventually produces bile ducts, the primary cystic duct exits the liver at the portal notch and transports the bile to the gall bladder where it is stored and concentrated.

The blood supply of the liver is provided by the hepatic artery and the hepatic portal vein from the intestines. The blood from each of these mixes within the lobules before exiting the liver via hepatic veins directly into the caudal vena cava embedded in the margin of the liver.

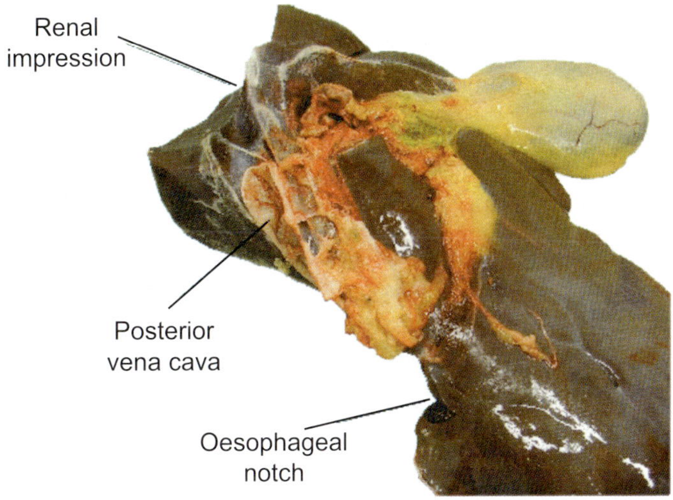

Bovine liver

BILE

This is produced by the hepatocytes and is a complex formula of water, pigments (biliverdin and bilirubin), fats, minerals and bile salts the latter being produced from cholesterol by organelles within the hepatocytes. The bile salts are saponification agents, they react with the fat in food allowing it to be further broken down by lipase. Bile salts are reabsorbed in the area of the ileum, bile pigments colour the faeces brown after conversion to urobilinogen by microbial action in the intestines.

FUNCTIONS OF THE LIVER

In addition to the production of bile, the liver can be considered the chemical and filtration organ of the body.

- It receives absorbed food for further processing or storage via the hepatic portal circulation where it converts short chain fatty acids into longer chain fatty acids either to be used immediately or stored within the liver. Glycogen is stored after conversion of glucose for recombination and release into the bloodstream. In addition lactic acid formed during muscular activity is taken to the liver for recombination to glucose for immediate use or glycogen for storage.
- Essential amino acids from the body are combined within the hepatocytes to produce proteins.

- Most plasma proteins are produced within the liver, including those that assist in the regulation of blood volume.
- Essential blood clotting factors including fibrinogen are produced in the liver.
- Urea is produced in the liver after protein deamination and enters the bloodstream to be removed by the kidneys.
- The phagocytic properties of hepatic cells (Kupfer cells) remove bacteria and other invasive organisms from the blood including that of the hepatic portal circulation. This filtration system is important, the liver acts as a line of defence against infection borne through the digestive system ideally purifying the blood before it is returned to the circulation proper.

CARDIOVASCULAR SYSTEM

INTRODUCTION

The cardiovascular system refers to the heart, blood and blood vessels. This represents a sealed system of tubes through which a fluid media (blood) is pumped by the heart. The cardiovascular system can be considered the transportation system of the body, carrying items to the tissue cells of the body including food, messages and protection, and removing the waste products of their existence.

BLOOD

This is a high viscosity red fluid, consisting of a fluid part (plasma) and cellular elements, that clots rapidly on exposure to air. Plasma is a straw coloured, protein rich fluid containing water, salts, nutrients, waste products of cellular metabolism and hormones. Suspended within this fluid is the cellular portion, red and white corpuscles and platelets.

The red corpuscles, erythrocytes, are biconcave discs with a thin capsular membrane with extensions that enter the cell forming a fine internal lattice, and are distinctive in that they possess no nucleus. The membranous lattice enmeshes haemoglobin, a protein that readily converts to oxyhaemoglobin in the presence of oxygen in the lungs and transports this oxygen to the cell tissues where it is released in return for the carbon dioxide waste of the cells which binds to the haemoglobin until returned to the lungs.

The white corpuscles, leucocytes, form part of the immune system recognising and digesting foreign material including bacteria, neutralising toxins and removing dead or damaged tissue. The platelets possess no nucleus and form part of the clotting mechanism.

BLOOD VESSELS

The blood vessels carry the blood throughout the body, arteries carrying blood under pressure from the heart, veins carrying blood back to the heart. The arteries have a three layered wall, an inner wall (*tunica interna*) of endothelial cells on an elastic connective tissue membrane, a central layer (*tunica media*) comprised of smooth muscle and elastic tissue, and a fibrous outer layer (*tunica adventitia*) that provides a defence against overexpansion of the arterial wall and possible rupture. This layering allows for expansion of the artery during the pump phase of the hearts movement (systole) followed by elastic relaxation and return to normal size during the rest phase, an action which also serves to further propel the blood along the artery. The arteries branch to smaller diameter arterioles which in turn branch into capillaries from which they are differentiated by retaining a proportion of muscle in their walls to regulate blood flow. The capillaries are thin tubes of endothelial cells on a thin connective tissue support, allowing fluid to leave the blood at the arterial end of the capillary bed to 'bathe' the tissue cells before a percentage of this fluid re-enters toward the venous portion of the capillary bed. The capillaries then reform into venuoles and then veins for return to the heart. The veins are thinner walled than arteries as they do not suffer the effects of the systolic 'pump', the muscular *tunica media* being confined to the larger veins. The *tunica interna* is thinner but forms one way valves within the vein to prevent back flow of the low pressure blood.

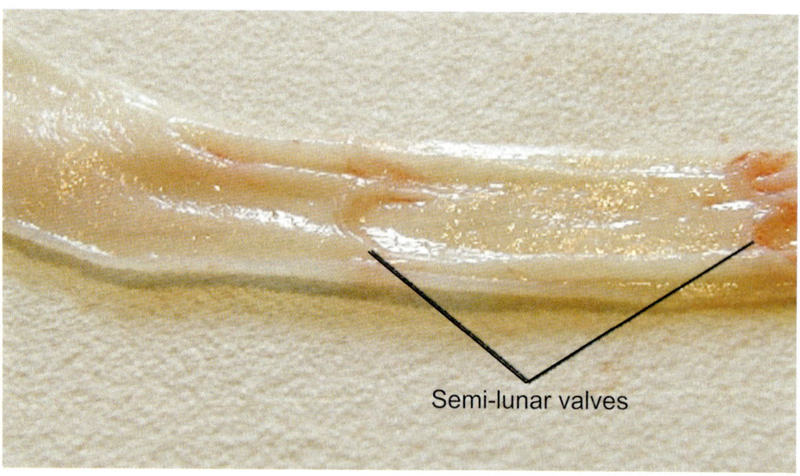

Semi-lunar valves in a dissected femoral vein

THE HEART

APPEARANCE

The bovine heart is a muscular organ, roughly conical in appearance consisting of four chambers - the right auricle and ventricle and the left auricle and ventricle, each side separated by a septum. The left side of the heart has thicker muscular walls and supplies arterial blood to the body under pressure. The ventricles are divided from the atria by valves (bicuspid between the left ventricle and auricle, tricuspid between the right ventricle and auricle), these valves are prevented from inverting under pressure by tendons, *Chordae tendineae*, that originate from the endocardium (the membrane lining the cavities). The heart is enclosed in a serous sac, the pericardium, which is an invagination of the parietal pleura that secretes fluid to both nourish and lubricate the heart as it beats. The pericardium itself has a visceral and parietal layer, the visceral pericardium being attached to the surface of the heart forming the epicardium, the parietal pericardium containing more fibrin.

CARDIAC MUSCLE

The heart muscle, cardiac muscle, is a specialised form of musculature. As with skeletal muscle it appears striated microscopically and contains the sarcomeres associated with skeletal muscle. Cardiac muscle is differentiated from skeletal muscle tissue in unique ways; the two main differences are by-products of the method of function of the heart muscle. Firstly the cardiac muscle is formed by single cells containing a single nucleus as opposed to the multi-nucleated fusion of myoblasts that form skeletal muscle. The second notable difference is that the myofibrils of actin and myosin are branched in cardiac muscle and interlock with those of adjacent fibres to form immensely strong junctions that prevent the fibres separating during the forceful contractions associated with a heart beat.

The contraction of the heart muscle is set up by the fibres themselves, the contraction of one sarcomere initialising contraction of its neighbour via gap junctions, thereby creating a wave effect of contraction starting at the auricle and proceeding down the ventricle forcing blood from the heart. The nervous supply to the heart simply offers only modulation of this beat either speed or strength. The table below illustrates the basic difference between cardiac and skeletal muscle.

Skeletal Muscle	Cardiac Muscle
Multi-nucleated, fusion of myoblasts	Single celled fibres, single nucleus
ATP derived from three sources, creatine phosphate, glycogen, and cellular respiration	ATP almost exclusively via cellular respiration, thus more mitochondria
Myofibrils separated	Myofibrils branched and interlocked
Motor nerve stimulates contraction	Motor nerve modulates contraction
Glycogen stores ten times larger than quantity of ATP stored	Small amount of glycogen stored

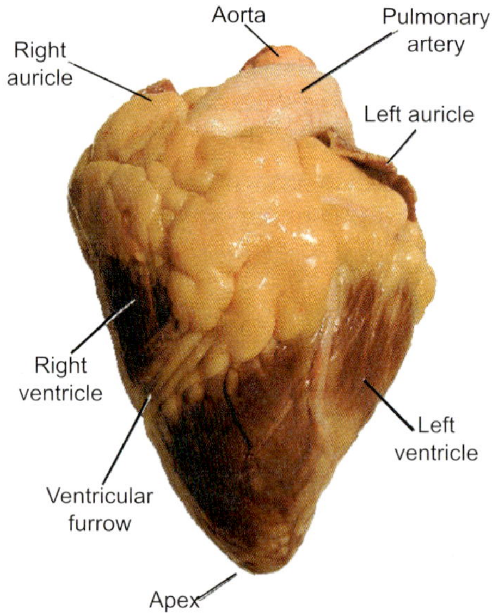

Bovine heart

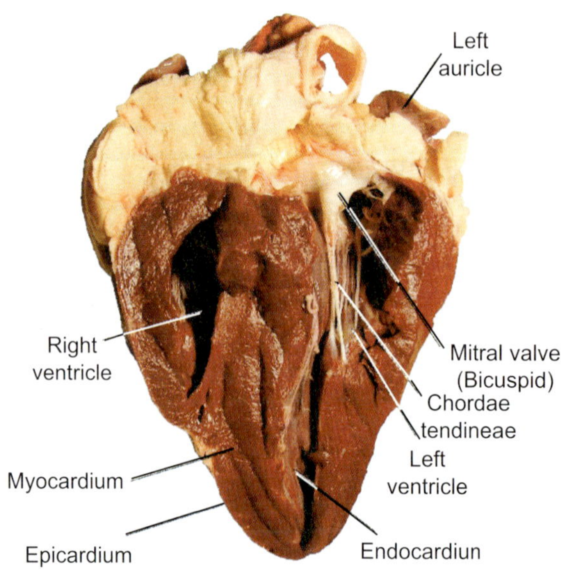

Dissected bovine heart

BLOOD CIRCULATION

The circulation of the blood throughout the body can be subdivided into three stages or circuits, the pulmonary circulation, the systemic circulation and the portal circulation.

Pulmonary Circulation

This system provides for the reoxygenation of the blood. Blood is pumped from the right ventricle via the pulmonary artery which bifurcates to enter each of the lung lobes where further subdivision of the arteries to arterioles and capillaries occurs. Once gaseous exchange takes place the pulmonary capillaries unite to form veins to take the purified blood back to the left auricle of the heart.

Systemic Circulation

The oxygenated blood then passes from the left auricle to the left ventricle via the bicuspid valve and is pumped through the aorta from which arteries branch off followed by further subdivision into arterioles and capillaries conveying the blood to all the tissues of the body. These capillaries then reunite to form venuoles and veins which carry the impure deoxygenated blood back to the heart via the anterior and posterior vena cava.

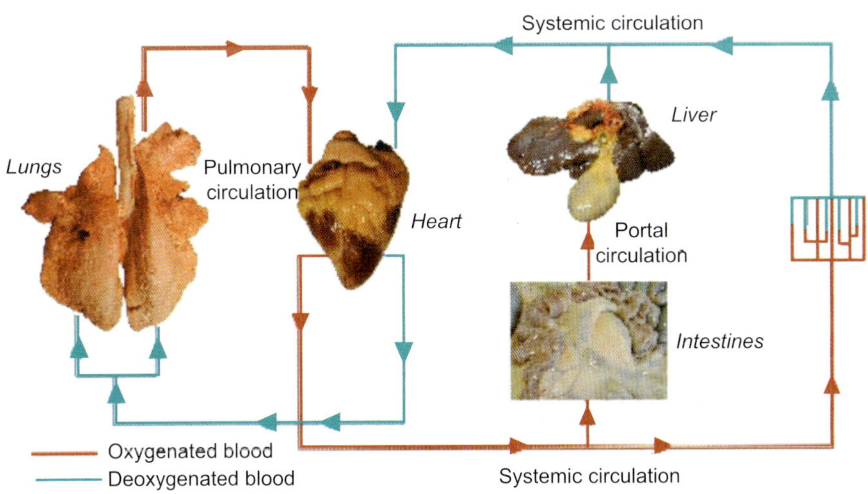

Portal Circulation

The portal circulation carries the blood from the intestines and stomachs to the liver via the portal vein. Once the blood has passed through the liver and the nutrients removed for conversion or added to the blood by the liver it passes into the normal circulation by being discharged into the posterior vena cava or via the hepatic vein back to the heart.

BLOOD CLOTTING

The clotting of blood is achieved by the action of platelets in conjunction with the protein fibrinogen which is carried in the plasma. On exposure to air platelets bind together and release thrombokinase. Thrombokinase reacts with prothrombin, produced by the liver, and plasma calcium to produce the enzyme thrombin which then converts fibrinogen to fibrin. The filamentous fibrin then forms a lattice of insoluble material that enmeshes corpuscles to form a clot. Blood serum is plasma from which fibrinogen has been removed during clotting.

THE LYMPHATIC SYSTEM

LYMPH VESSELS

These are thin walled, blind-ended tubes that operate in association with the blood circulatory system of blood vessels and capillary beds. The fluid they contain performs the function of bathing the tissue cells providing them with nutrients, hormones and oxygen before removing carbon dioxide and waste material back to the blood stream. The blood capillaries of the area remove the majority of the carbon dioxide; particulate matter is taken up by the tissue fluid and removed to the lymphatic circulation. Circulation of lymph through the vessels is mainly due to contraction of surrounding muscle beds. The lymph vessels converge into two larger ducts which discharge the fluid back into the blood stream at the jugular veins, the right duct joining the right jugular and the left, or thoracic duct joining the left jugular vein. The thoracic duct is dilated at the point where the smaller vessels converge to form the *cisterna chyli* (*receptaculum chyli*).

LYMPH

This is a fluid, similar to blood plasma that enters the lymphatic system. It contains significantly less protein than blood plasma and as a consequence is less viscous and able to move in and out of the vessels easily.

LYMPH NODES

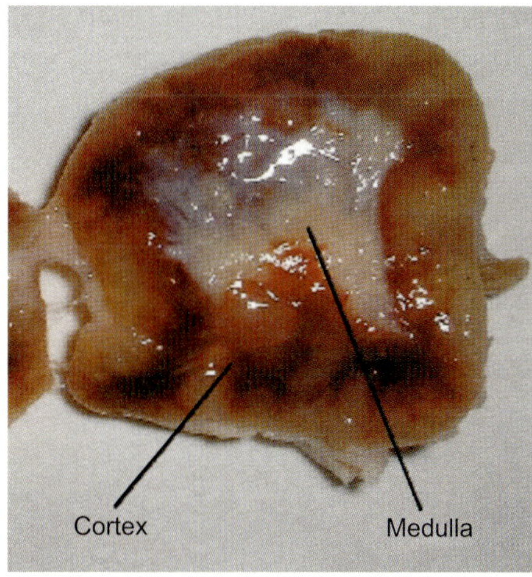

The bovine body has lymph nodes situated at specific points, each one acting as a filter for lymph fluid drained from a particular area and as such the change of state of a node is an indicator of infection in that drainage area. Therefore knowledge of the position and normal appearance of these nodes and their respective drainage areas is of the utmost importance to the meat inspector.

Before returning to the blood circulation lymph fluid passes through at least one lymph node. These are accumulations of lymphoid material encapsulated within a connective tissue shell, forming a firm oval, or more generally bean shaped node. The lymph entering a node is termed afferent lymph; that leaving the node is termed the efferent lymph. Lymph nodes consist of two regions; the medulla and cortex, each of these regions has a specific function. The cortex contains germinal centres in which continual lymphocyte production takes place, and the medulla contains a lattice containing phagocytic cells. The lymph fluid enters the capsule through afferent vessels entering the surface of the node and into the sub capsular sinus, the fluid then percolates through the cortical region collecting more lymphocytes and then through the medulla where any foreign particular matter, including bacteria is removed by phagocytosis before the lymph leaves the node through the efferent vessels situated at the hilus of the node.

POSITION OF NODES AND DRAINAGE AREAS

Head

Node	Position	Afferent	Efferent
Parotid	Ventral to mandibular joint, overlying masseter muscle	Dorsal half of the head	Lateral retropharyngeal

Head (Contd)

Node	Position	Afferent	Efferent
Submaxillary	Medial to mandible	Nasal mucosa and ventral area of the head including larynx	Lateral retropharyngeal
Retropharyn-geal	Dorsal to pharynx medial to long horn of hyoid bone	Deep tissues of the head	Lateral retropharyngeal

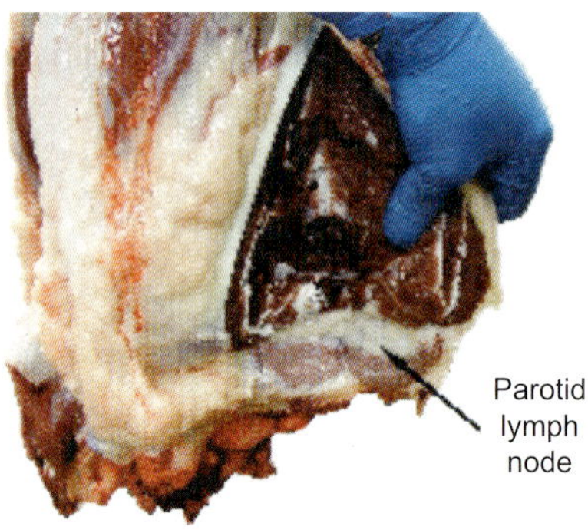

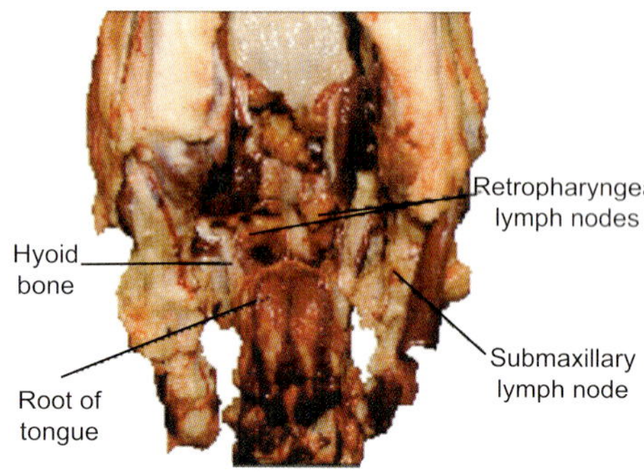

Abdominal Viscera

Node	Position	Afferent	Efferent
Mesenteric nodes	Chain from duodenum to caecum in fat of mesentery	Jejunum and ileum	Cisterna chyli or local lymph trunks
Renal	In fat at hilus of kidney	Kidneys	Cisterna chyli
Hepatic portal	On visceral surface of liver in area of portal vein and hepatic artery	Liver, pancreas and duodenum	Intestinal lymph trunks and mediastinal nodes

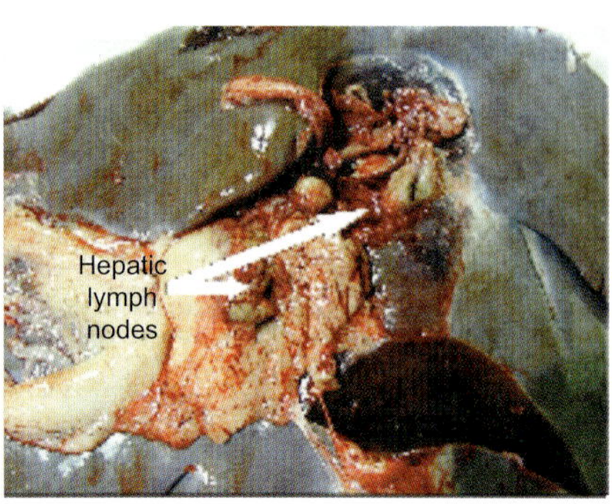

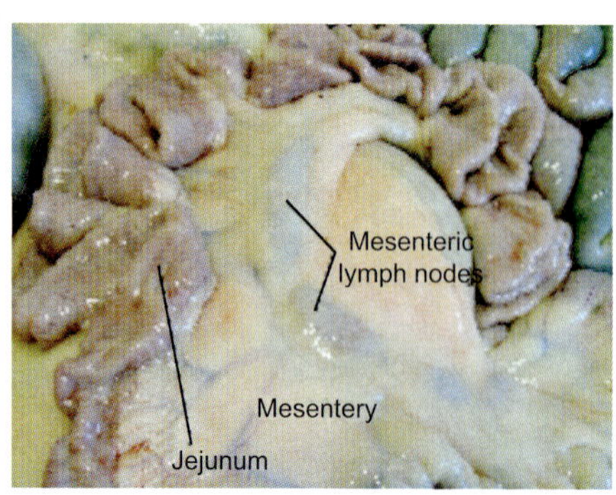

Lungs

Node	Position	Afferent	Efferent
Bronchial	Caudal to the bifurcation of the trachea	Trachea, heart, pulmonary and thoracic aortic nodes	Mediastinal nodes or thoracic duct
Mediastinal	Chain of nodes running from in fat cranial to heart down the oesophagus to caudal to the heart	Mediastinal tissue, diaphragm, spleen, liver, parietal pleura and intercostals, bronchial and aortic nodes	Cervical nodes

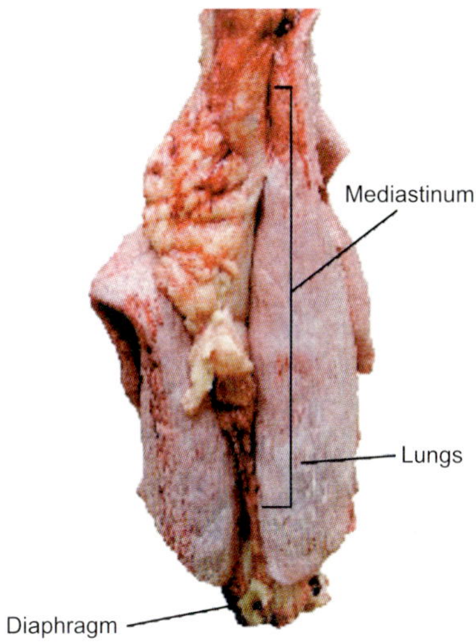

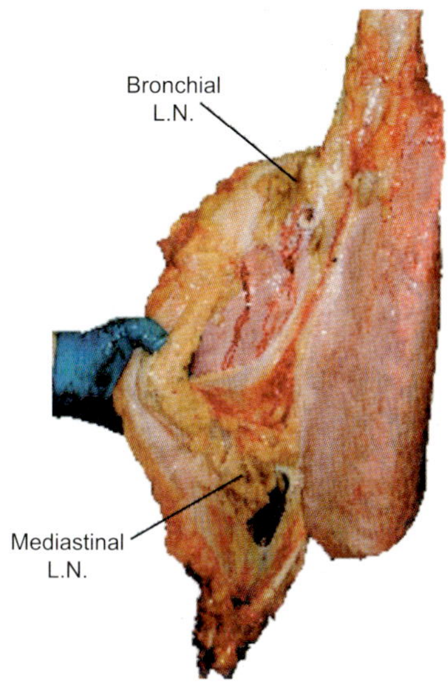

Neck

Node	Position	Afferent	Efferent
Lateral retropharyn-geal	Ventral to wing of the atlas bone	Caudal head, cranial neck, parotid and submaxillary nodes	Forms the tracheal duct
Deep cervical	Close to trachea and oesophagus	Local tissues	Tracheal trunk

Forelimb

Node	Position	Afferent	Efferent
Prescapular	On cranial border of the supraspinatus muscle. Found by cutting approx 15cm deep by 5cm long.	Local tissues, head nodes, forelimb and cranial mammary glands	Cervical nodes

Forelimb (Contd)

Node	Position	Afferent	Efferent
Axillary	In the second intercostals space 6-10cm caudal to the shoulder joint	Local tissues of the shoulder and 'forearm'	Deep cervical

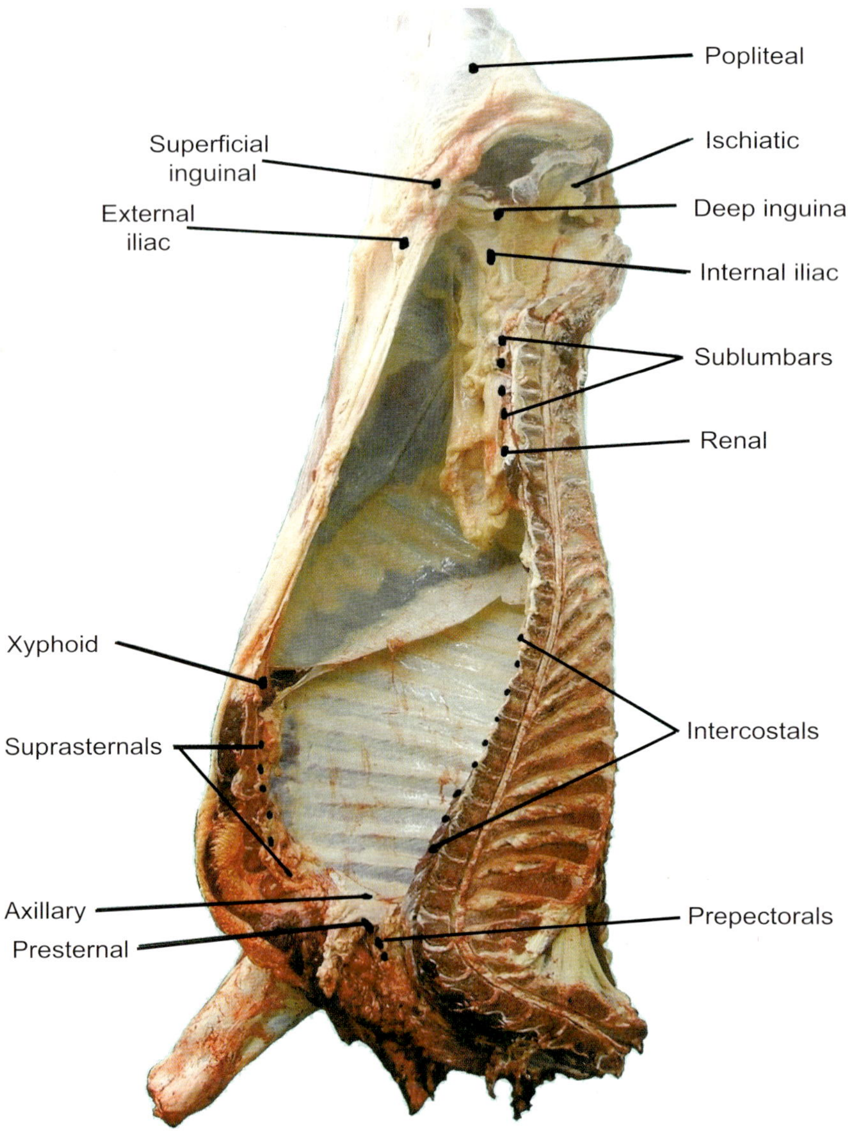

Lymph nodes of the bovine carcase – internal view

Thorax

Node	Position	Afferent	Efferent
Intercostal	In intercostal spaces at the level of the rib heads	Chest wall, diaphragm and vertebrae	Mediastinal and thoracic aortic nodes
Sub dorsal (thoracic)	Dorsal border of aorta and T5-T13 vertebrae	Shoulder region, chest wall, diaphragm, heart, spleen, pleura and peritoneum, mediastinum, and intercostals and mediastinal nodes	Thoracic duct
Presternal	Ventral border of internal thoracic vessels level with first costal cartilage	Ventral chest wall, mediastinum, diaphragm	Thoracic and tracheal trunk
Suprasternal & Xiphoid	Along course of internal thoracic vessels	Diaphragm, pericardium, chest wall, liver, pectoral and abdominal muscles	Cranial sternal nodes

Abdomen

Node	Position	Afferent	Efferent
Sublumbar	Chain of small nodes each side of aorta and caudal vena cava	Lumbar region, abdominal wall, iliac nodes	Lumbar trunks and cisterna chyli
Internal iliac	Ventral to psoas minor muscles	Caudal half of abdominal wall, pelvic limb, urogenitalia, and superficial inguinal, popliteal and external iliac nodes	Lumbar trunks to cisterna chyli
External iliac	Either side of the bifurcation of the deep circumflex iliac vessels	Abdomen, deep gluteal and tensor fasciae latae muscles, peritoneum and sub iliac nodes	Lumbar aortic and internal iliac nodes
Superficial inguinal (male) Supramammary (female)	Male: Scrotal nodes between cod fat and abdominal wall. Female: Usually in a straight line with the cut pubic tubercle	External genitalia, abdominal wall, skin of hind limb and the udder in females	Internal iliac nodes
Ischiatic	Near sciatic nerve. Exposed by a deep incision through the middle gluteal muscle on a vertical line midway between the sacrum and the caudal part of the ischium	Pelvic and hip regions and popliteal node	Internal iliac nodes

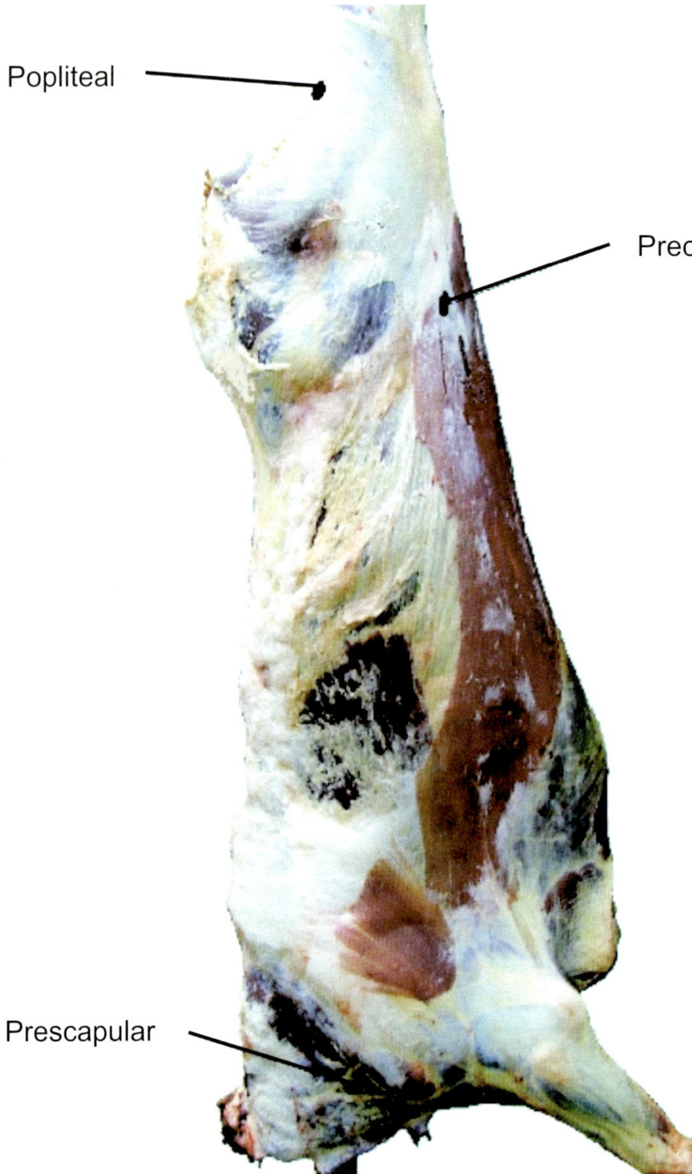

Lymph nodes of the bovine carcase – external view

Hindlimb

Node	Position	Afferent	Efferent
Precrural	Midway between patella and *tuber coxae* of ilium	Thigh, abdominal wall, umbilicus and caudal part of thorax	Iliac nodes
Popliteal	Caudal to stifle joint, found by separating biceps and semitend-onosus muscles	Distal limb	Internal iliac and ischiatic nodes

LYMPHOID TISSUE

Lymphoid tissue also forms part of the lymphoid system; however it is not as formalised and discrete as lymph nodes. Lymphoid tissue is found throughout the body such as in the liver and in the bronchi of the lungs and represents a method of localised response to pathogenic particles. Lymphoid tissue is primarily a latticework of tissue containing interspatial lymphocytes. The accumulation of the tissue tends to be in areas where infectious organisms may gain entry into the body, most noticeably amongst these is the lymphoid tissue of the digestive system, the gut associated lymphoid tissue (GALT) including the tonsils, the connective tissue layer of the mucous membrane of the intestines, and the Peyer's patches; the latter of which are recognised as raised oval shaped areas in the mucosal and sub mucosal layers of the lower intestine.

THE SPLEEN

The spleen, also known as the 'melt' in cattle, is a mottled greyish-blue organ that is thin, flat and ovoid in shape. In life it is positioned in the upper left hand side of the abdominal cavity attached to the rumen by the omentum. It consists of a firm capsule enclosing red and white pulp into which the capsule extends forming a supporting network called trabeculae. The spleen is supplied by the splenic artery which branches from the celiac artery. The white pulp can be observed when the spleen is incised and represents areas of lymphoid tissue aggregated near the arteries that pass through the spleen. These areas of white pulp (Malphigian corpuscles) possess lymphogenic and phagocytic properties, removing old and diseased red blood cells and particulate matter from the circulation in addition to adding lymphocytes to the blood leaving the spleen via the splenic vein to the portal vein.

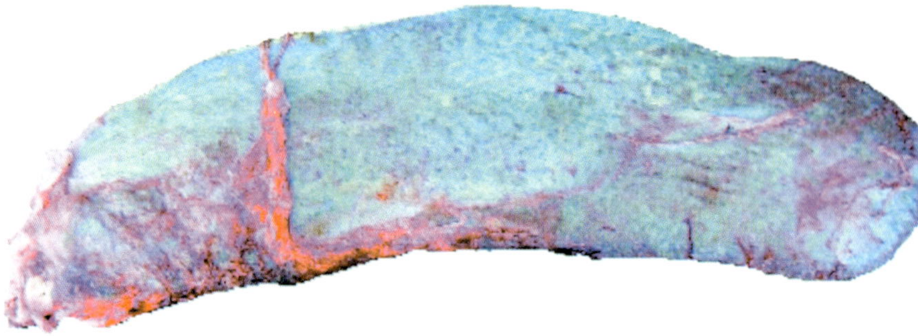

Bovine Spleen

The red pulp acts as a blood storage reservoir in addition to the production of erythrocytes, the latter function utilising the iron stored in the spleen after the destruction of damaged erythrocytes by the white pulp.

The splenic capsule and substance is innervated by nerves entering with the artery, and possesses the ability to contract forcing stored blood into the circulation in times of need.

UROGENITAL SYSTEM

URINARY TRACT

INTRODUCTION

The deamination of proteins in the liver releases toxic nitrogenous compounds that are subsequently converted to urea and released into the blood circulation. The main function of the urinary system is the filtration of toxic substances including urea from the blood and then excreting them from the body. This filtration and excretion system consists of paired kidneys, paired ureters, a bladder and a single urethra.

KIDNEY STRUCTURE

Bovine kidneys consist of 15-20 chocolate brown coloured lobes, each acting as an individual kidney. Both kidneys are embedded in thick renal fat in a position lateral to the vertebrae. The right kidney is held tight against the body, the left has a looser attachment enabling movement of the organ in relation to the expansion of the rumen thereby preventing the kidney from being crushed, the left kidney is also characterised by a slight rotation about its axis. The kidneys are further covered by a membranous renal capsule that can be easily peeled in the healthy animal.

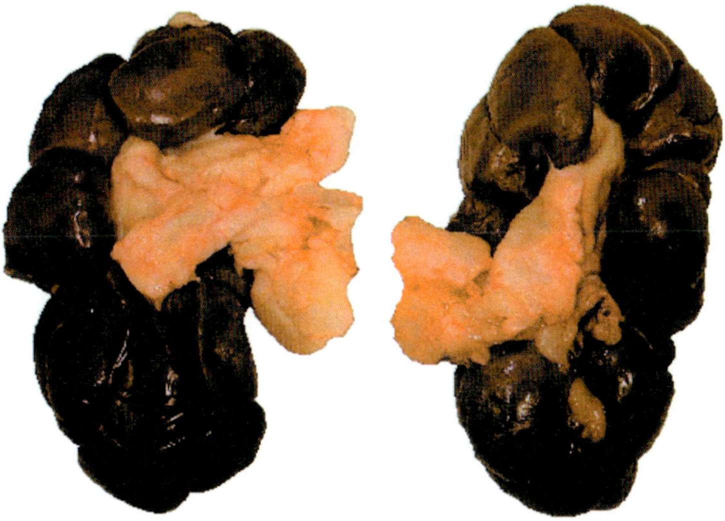

Left and right bovine kidneys

In cross section each lobe of the kidney is found to contain a cortex, medulla, calyx and renal pelvis, the latter of which forms the ureter.

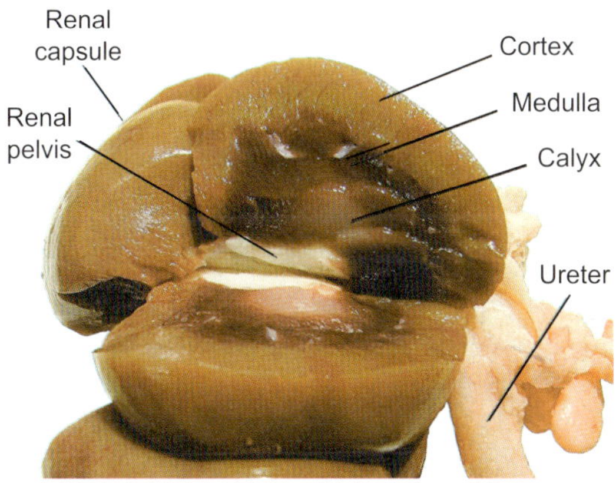

Dissection of a kidney lobule

The renal cortex contains nephrons, each comprising a glomerus and tubule in units known as Malphigian bodies. The glomerus is basically a knot of blood capillaries surrounded by a capsule (Bowman's capsule). One side of the capsule joins a collecting tubule that is surrounded by blood capillaries. The tubule, at first convoluted, extends down into the medulla before returning back to the cortex, the loop of the tubule in the medulla being the loop of Henlé.

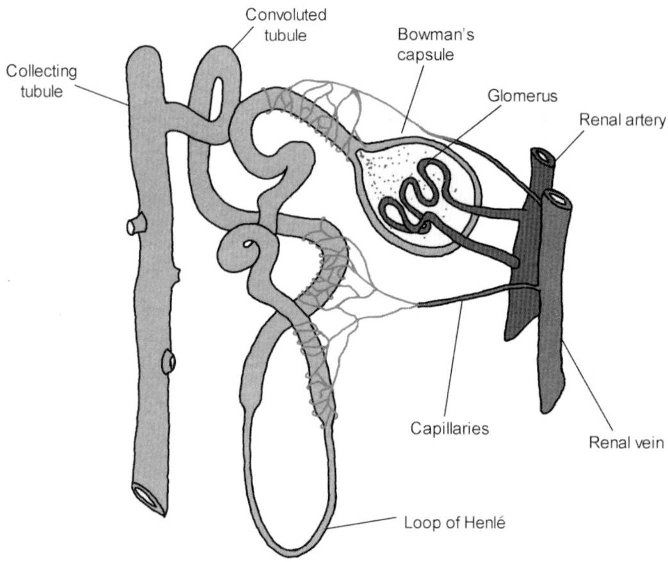

Schematic of a nephron. Bowman's capsule peeled to show glomerus.

FUNCTION OF THE KIDNEY

Blood at arterial pressure enters the glomerus which forces the fluid portion of the blood into the Bowman's capsule. This fluid then moves down the tubule during which time the majority is reabsorbed into the capillaries that surround it. Approximately 20% of the fluid and the urea etc remains to enter the main collecting tubule to trickle into the renal pelvis.

URETERS

The renal pelvis is formed by the expanded ureter, down which the urine trickles into the bladder. The ureter is a thin walled tube with a coat of fibrous tissue surrounding a layer of involuntary muscle and an internal mucous membrane. The ureters pass along the body of the bladder before discharging near its' neck.

BLADDER

The bladder is a pear shaped distensible sac that possesses a similar wall structure to the ureters and is situated on the pubic bone but when full extends

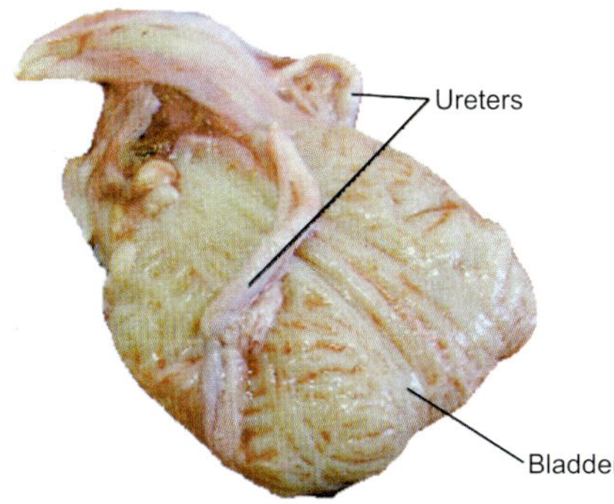

into the abdominal cavity under the peritoneum. The control of urine entering the bladder is physical; as the bladder expands it exerts pressure on the ureters as they pass over its' body and reduce the flow of urine into the bladder. This action also has the effect of preventing reflux of urine from the bladder into the ureters. The neck of the bladder contains a ring of involuntary sphincter muscle which in conjunction with an external skeletal sphincter muscle under conscious control of the animal regulates the flow of urine into the urethra.

URETHRA

A single urethra emanates from the neck of the bladder and follows the floor of the pelvis to which it is held by fat and connective tissue. In the female the urethra is short; the dorsal surface is also attached to the outer wall of the vagina into which it discharges in the vestibule ventral to the hymen. In males the urethra consists of a pelvic and a penile area, continuing to the tip of the penis.

REPRODUCTIVE SYSTEM

FEMALE REPRODUCTIVE SYSTEM

INTRODUCTION

The reproductive system of the female bovine has specific functions; to produce the macrogametocyte (the ova or eggs to provide 50% of the genetic material of the calf), to provide an environment and opportunity for fertilisation of the egg, to provide a safe environment for the development and nutritional needs of the growing foetus and to provide a means of expelling the calf once developed by parturition (birth).

The female reproductive system, consisting of paired ovaries, paired oviducts (uterine horns), single uterus, single cervix and single vagina, lie parallel and ventral to the rectum, being attached to this by membrane and fat. The reproductive system terminates externally at the vulva.

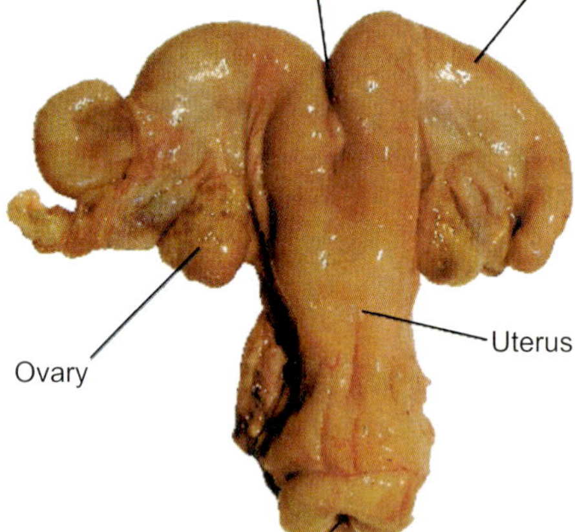

Female reproductive tract

OVARIES

There are two ovaries (left and right) whose functions include the formation of eggs and the secretion of the hormones oestrogen and progesterone. Eggs are produced and matured in primordial follicles; water filled cavities within the ovary consisting of an outer layer of oestrogen producing cells.

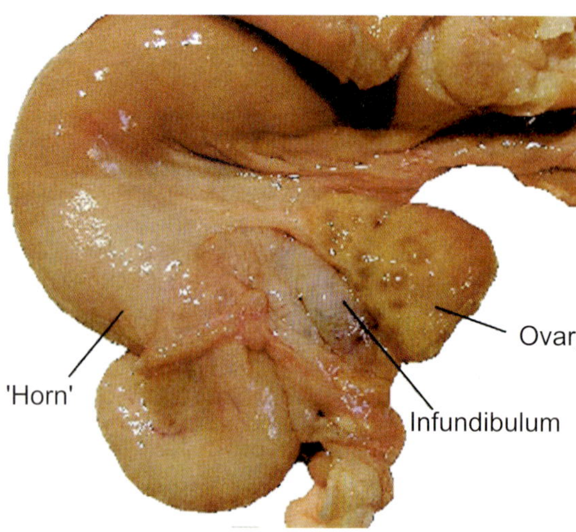

The formation of these cyst-like bodies (follicles) and the subsequent maturation of the eggs is stimulated by Follicle Stimulating Hormone (FSH) produced within the pituitary gland. The levels of a second hormone also produced in the pituitary gland, Lutenizing

Hormone (LH) stimulates the secretion of oestrogen by the follicle cells and finally prompts the release of the ovum from the follicle (ovulation) after the follicle ripens into a mature cyst known as a Graafian follicle.

Once the ovum has left the ruptured follicle, the latter degenerates into a yellowish glandular mass, the *corpus luteum*, which secretes progesterone, a hormone that aids implantation of a fertilised ovum within the uterus. If conception does not occur the *corpus luteum* regresses and a new follicle forms. If conception occurs the *corpus luteum* regresses in the latter stages of the pregnancy to be replaced by white fibrous tissue at which point it is termed the *corpus albicans*.

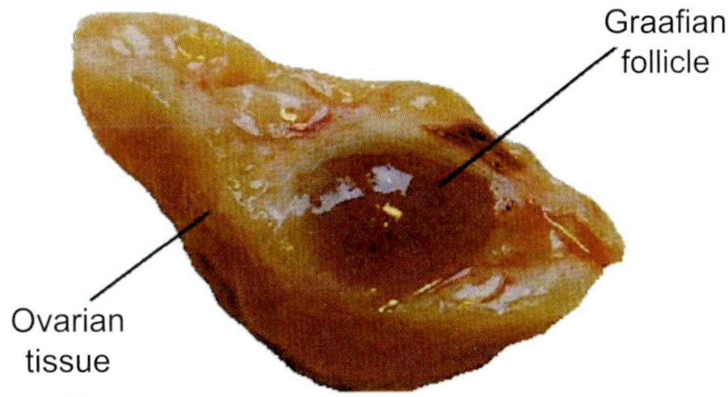

UTERINE HORNS

These paired structures are embedded in a uterine ligament which holds them in position against the ileum. The ovaries are surrounded by finger-like projections of the funnel shaped infundibulum designed to guide released ova into the body of the uterine horns which join to form a single uterine body. The uterus and uterine horns are comprised of an internal mucosal membrane(endometrium) containing glands whose size varies with the stage of the reproductive cycle, a muscular wall (myometrium) of both inner circular and outer longitudinal muscles the contractions of which at parturition expel the calf, and a final outer membrane (perimetrium) that is formed by the uterine ligament.

The endometrium also serves as the site of attachment of the maternal side of the placenta, the position of which is determined by the presence of up to 100 cotyledons, circular vallate structures approximately 5-10mm diameter in the non-pregnant heifer but expanding during pregnancy.

CERVIX

The cervix represents the terminus of the uterus, a cervical canal surrounded by five muscular rings that in conjunction with a mucous plug form an impervious sphincter that relaxes during oestrus to allow sperm to pass through and dilates at parturition to allow the calf to be born.

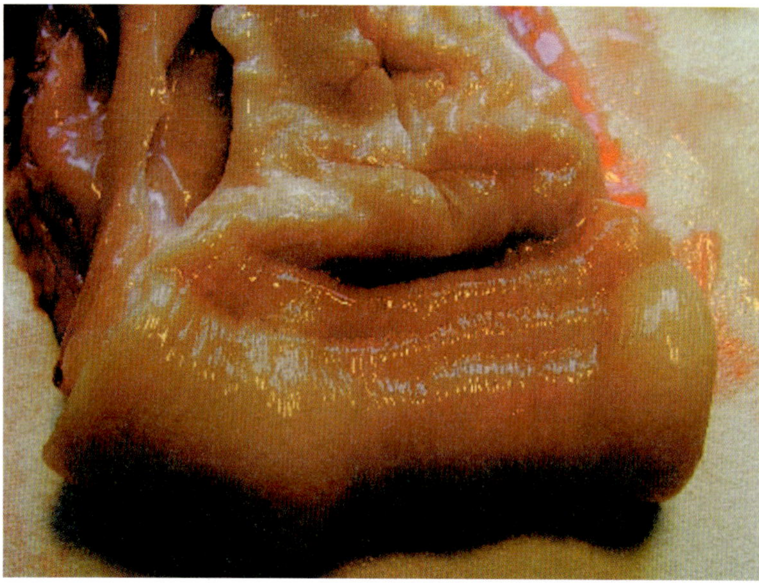

A dissected cervix, illustrating the banding of the muscle

THE VAGINA

The vagina starts at the cervical canal and terminates at the vulva. It has a highly elastic structure and lies in the pelvis and is attached dorsally to the ventral surface of the rectum. In addition to being the site at which the urethra terminates at the external urethral orifice on the floor of the vagina, the vagina accepts the penis and sperm from the male during copulation.

MAMMARY GLANDS

The mammary glands are modified sweat glands containing connective tissue, blood vessels, lymphatic vessels and glandular tissue. Alveoli within the gland tissue secrete and store milk which is then collected in ducts and delivered to the teats. Cattle possess four mammary glands each with a teat, combined to form the udder. The udder is visibly separated into two halves along the median plane by the presence of suspensory sheets; the division between the two glands on each side of the separation is indistinct as the glandular tissue of one gland tends to fuse with that of the other. The milk produced collects in interconnecting ducts before entering the teat cistern. The teat contains a single duct usually held closed by a combination of the naturally elasticity of the connective tissue of the teat and an encircling layer of smooth muscle.

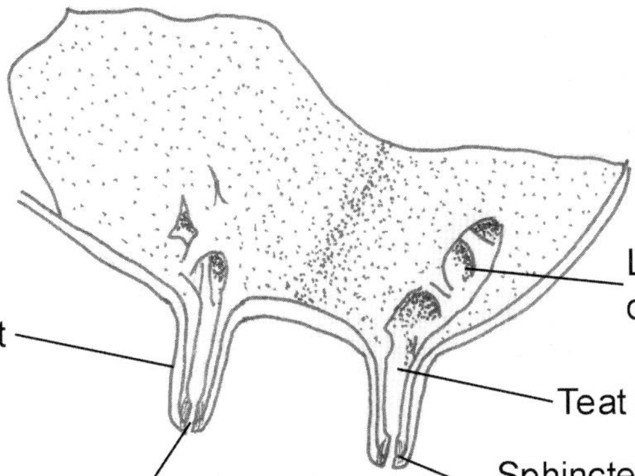

Diagrammatic cross section of a mammary gland

MALE REPRODUCTIVE SYSTEM

INTRODUCTION

The male reproductive system consists of paired testicles suspended in a scrotal sac, the penis, and glands such as the bulbourethral gland and the seminal vesicles. The function of these being to produce, mature and deliver half of the genetic material (spermatozoa) required to produce a foetus in conjunction with the female ova.

TESTES

A single bull's testicle weighs approximately 300g and is oval, the length generally being twice the breadth. These glandular organs hang in a scrotal sac formed by a fold in the abdomen between the hind legs of the bull. The internal surface of the scrotum is continuous with the peritoneum and is smooth and serosal. The paired testes are suspended in the scrotum by the spermatic cord which contains the red cremaster muscle enabling the testes to be individually raised or lowered in the scrotum in response to external temperatures (as the production of sperm is highly temperature dependant), in addition to the testicular artery and the pampiniform plexus (a convoluted series of the testicular veins that spiral around the artery). The *ductus deferens* that carries the spermatozoa to the urethra is attached to the visceral vaginal tunic that surrounds the spermatic cord.

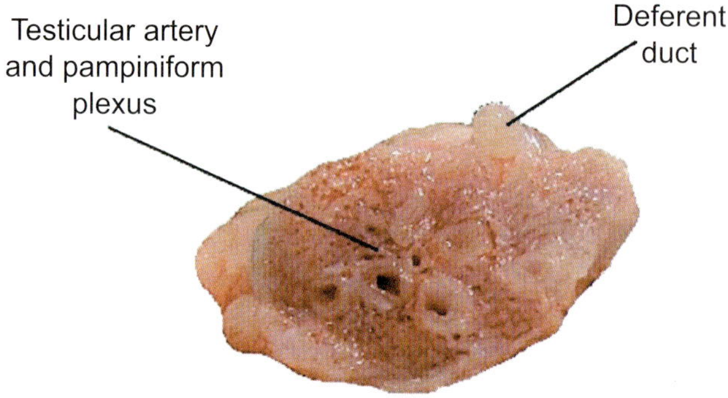

Transection of the spermatic cord

On the median line of each testicle is the epididymis, folded back on itself at each pole forming a semi-pyramidal extension to the base of the testicle as it hangs in the scrotal sac. The epididymis is recognised as having three zones, the head leaving the testicle, the body, and the tail, and provides storage for the maturation of sperm prior to ejaculation.

The *ductus deferens* also known as the *vas deferens* is the tubular continuation of the epididymis and provides the linkage between the epididymis and the urethra for the transportation of the sperm.

On dissection the testes are found to comprise a yellowish coloured lobulated substance formed by tightly coiled tubes called seminiferous tubules in which the sperm are produced, and leydig cells which secrete the hormone testosterone.

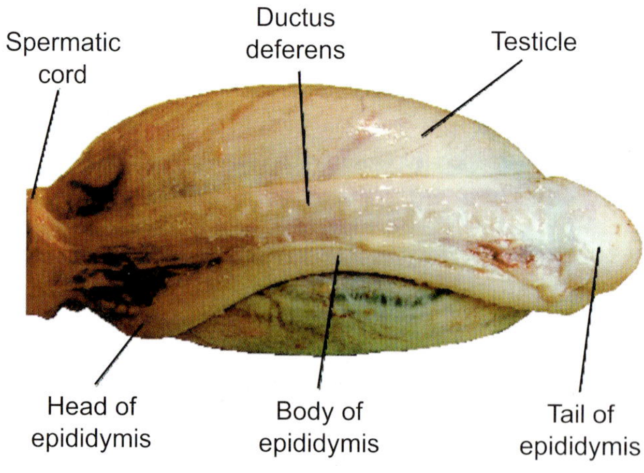

Bovine testicle

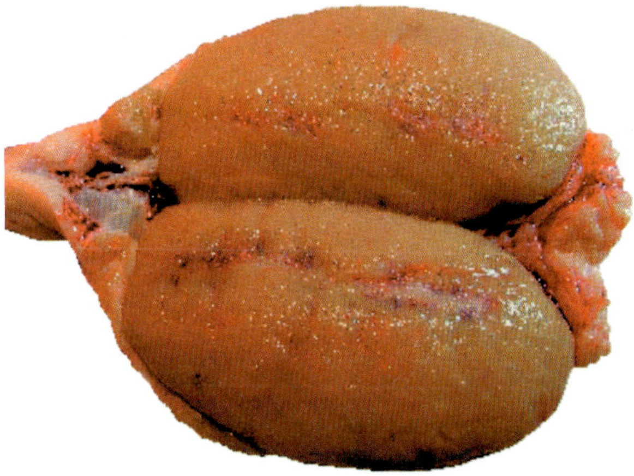

Dissection of a testicle along the median plane

URETHRA AND PENIS

The penis has a dual role, as a delivery system for semen during copulation and the expulsion of urine from the body, both functions utilising the urethra that extends from the neck of the urinary bladder to the tip of the penis. The *ductus deferens* from each testicle passes dorsally over the bladder at which point the mucosa of the duct is thickened by glandular cells to form the cylindrical ampullae which lie next to the lobulated vesicular glands, at which point the *ductus deferens* enter the urethra.

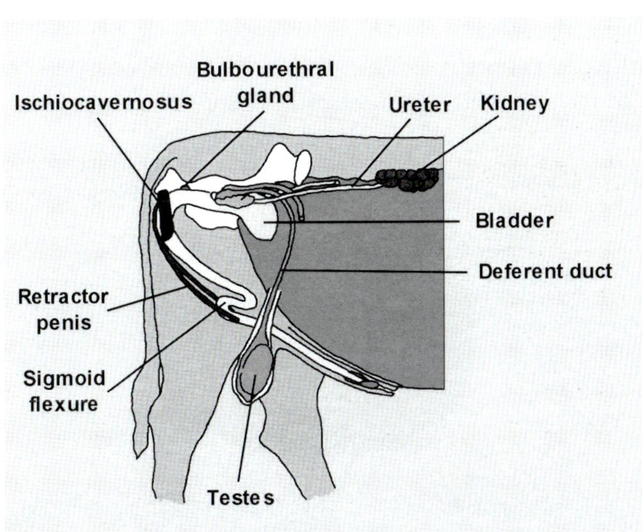

The pelvic urethra continues from the urinary bladder to the bulbourethral gland which adjoins the urethra via a small diverticulum. It is at this point the origin is situated of the *corpus cavernosum (ischiocavernosus)*, the column of erectile tissue that forms the main body of the penis. This origin, termed the crus penis is usually left near the ischial arch on the dressed carcase and can be used as a method of gender identification.

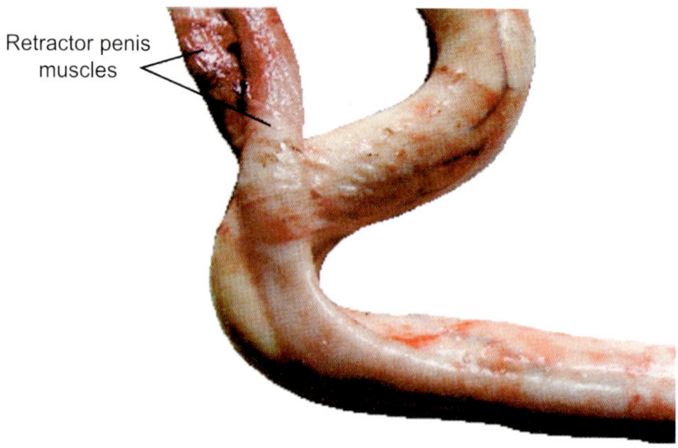

Detail of sigmoid flexure

The penis proper is composed of three columns of tissue with a rich arterial blood supply that surround the hollow urethra. Contained within a fibrous tunic (*Tunica albuginea*) and roughly circular in section, the dorsal aspect of the penis is formed by the two fused *corpus cavernosae* with the urethra surrounded by the *corpus spongiosum* carried in a ventral groove, the columns of *corpus cavernosae* terminate at the glans of the penis which is formed by the *corpus spongiosum*. In addition to the columns of erectile tissue the penis also contains a large proportion of connective tissue, and is characterised by the presence of a sigmoid flexure that straightens out when the penis becomes erect.

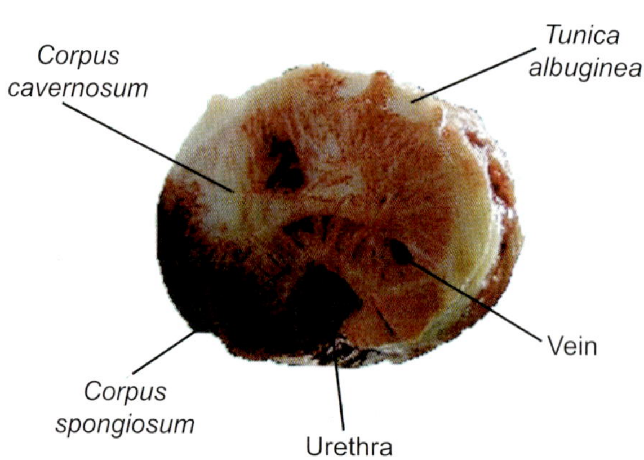

Transection of the penis, caudal to the sigmoid flexure

NERVOUS SYSTEM

INTRODUCTION

The nervous system is the body's messenger system, nerves prompting activities such as muscular action, organ activity and hormone secretion, as well as informing the brain of the condition of the body systems and the environment. The nervous system is divided into two regions, the Central Nervous System (the brain and spinal cord) and the Peripheral Nervous System (organs, muscles, skin etc.) These systems themselves function on two levels, the somatic nervous system, co-coordinating impulses that are under conscious control, and the autonomic system, controlling involuntary action such as heart beat, organ function and hormone secretion by glands.

NERVES

Nerves are non-microscopic, string like structures formed by bundled nerve cells that pass impulses between the central nervous system and parts or organs of the body. There are three basic forms of nerve, categorized by their function and the direction of the impulses, either from the central nervous system, to the central nervous system or both ways, these nerve types being efferent, sensory and intermediate. Efferent nerves (also known as motor nerves) transmit impulses from the central nervous system usually to groups of muscles, Sensory nerves convey impulses such as temperature or pain to the central nervous system and Intermediate nerves transmit impulses both ways.

NERVE CELLS

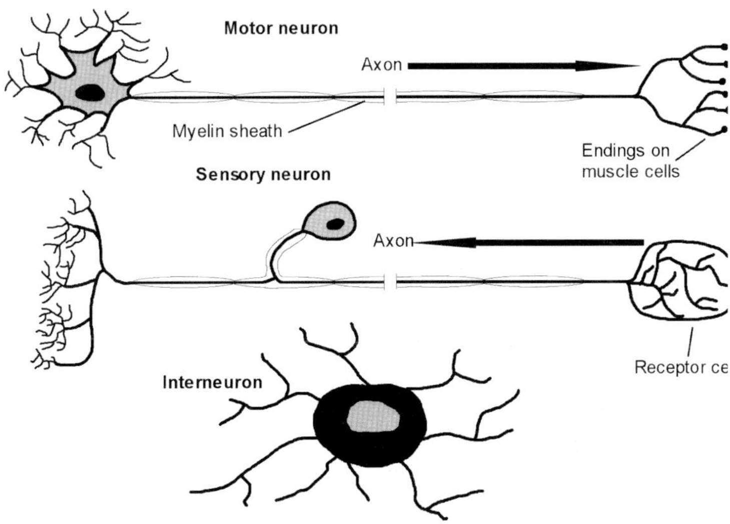

The nerve cell, or neuron, is the basis of the nervous system. The cell body is surrounded by dendrites, extensions of the cell wall, of which one is elongated to form the axon. During neuron development the axon is surrounded by specialist cells (Schwann cells) that spiral around the axon, this envelope of cells then secretes a layer of fat (myelin) forming an insulating sheath. Bundles of axons form the nerves, the sciatic nerve serving the hind leg contains axons of over a metre in length. The nerve chain forms circuits throughout the body, the cellular electrical impulse travelling along the axon from one nerve cell to the dendrite of another. Each nerve cell is separated from the next by a junction gap (synapse) across which chemical transmitters cross causing cellular excitement and a continuation of the impulse. Certain drugs including alcohol interfere with this system.

CENTRAL NERVOUS SYSTEM

The brain is situated in the cranial cavity of the skull and consists of two pear shaped hemispheres comprising the cerebrum and cerebellum. The base of the brain forms the medulla oblongata.

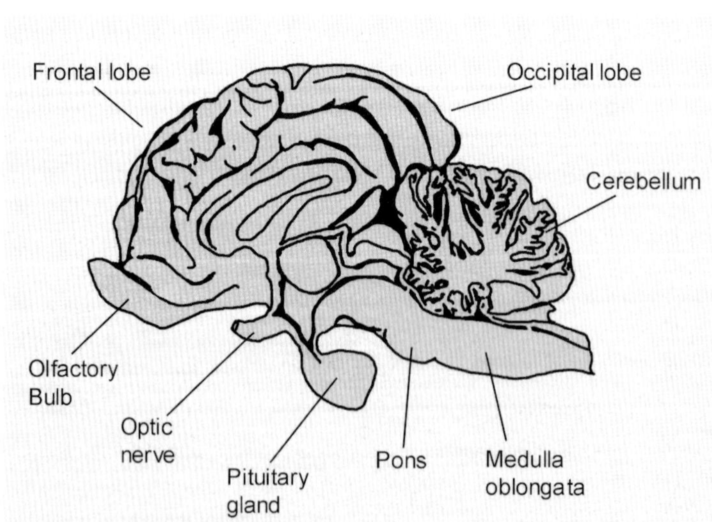

The spinal cord originates from the medulla oblongata and runs through a protective channel formed by the hollow mid-section of the spinal vertebrae down to the last free vertebrae of the tail.

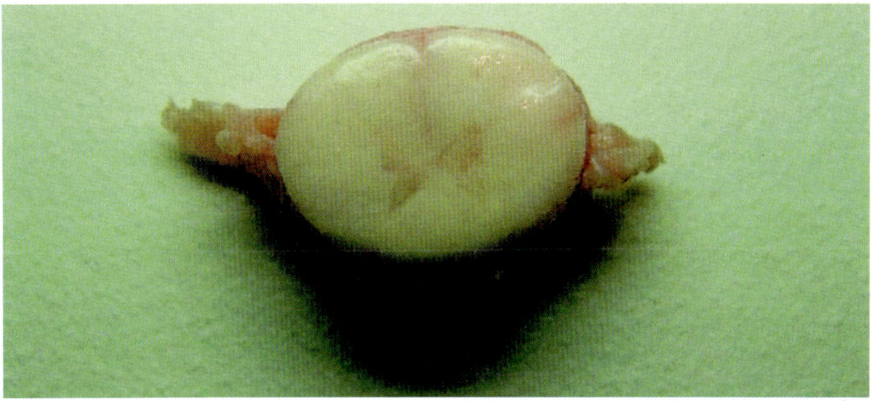

A cross section of the spinal cord

In cross section a 'butterfly' shaped area of grey matter can be seen surrounded by white matter. The grey matter is formed by interneurons; the white matter is created by the myelin sheath of the axons passing down the length of the spinal cord.

The spinal cord is covered by three layers of protective tissue, the meninges, consisting of the dura mater, a strong layer of connective tissue not attached to the periosteum of the spinal canal, the arachnoid mater, a fibrous layer with spaces containing the cerebrospinal fluid and the pia mater which provides nutrient and structural support to the neurons.

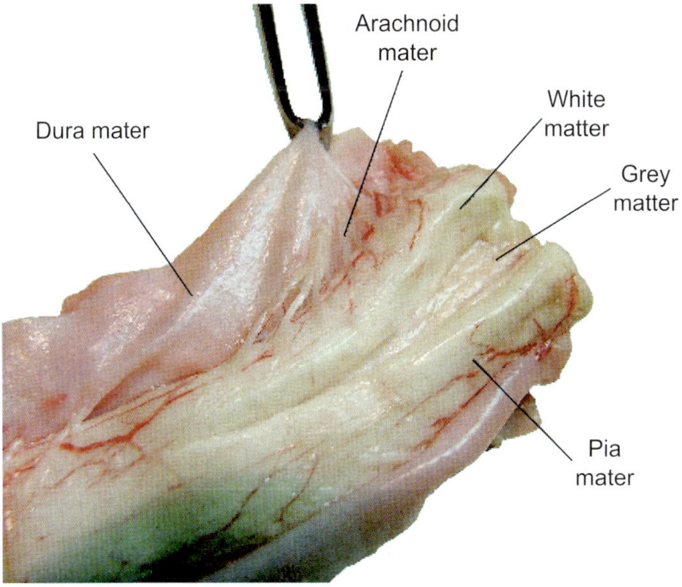

Dissection of the spinal cord meninges

PERIPHERAL NERVOUS SYSTEM

The peripheral nerves emanate symmetrically from each side of the spinal cord and pass through the body of the vertebrae. The nerves can be single or grouped together (plexus or ganglia). Two major groups of nerves are the brachial plexus, with nerves branching out to the forelimbs, which originates from the last four cervical and first thoracic vertebrae, and the sciatic or ischiadic nerve, the longest nerve in the body, which branches from the lumbrosacral plexus and runs down the thigh.

ENDOCRINE GLANDS

INTRODUCTION

Defined as the ductless glands, organs of the endocrine system possess specialist cells that secrete hormones (chemical transmitters used for communication and control within the body). These glands include the pituitary, thyroid, parathyroid, thymus, adrenals, pancreas and gonads.

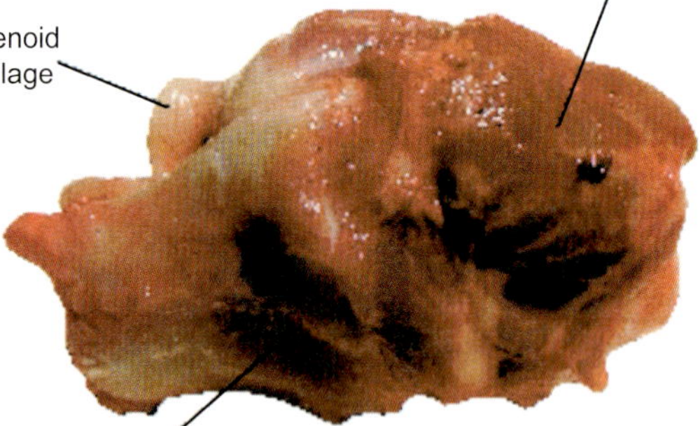

THYROID GLAND

This is a brownish gland situated on either side of the thyroid and cricoid cartilages of the larynx and joined on the dorsal surface by a narrow isthmus so that when removed it has been described as 'butterfly shaped.' It is composed of densely packed sacs containing a clear viscose fluid.

PARATHYROID GLAND

These are two to four pea sized glands lighter in colour to the thyroid glands in which they are embedded.

PITUITARY GLAND (HYPOPHYSIS)

This small yellowish-brown bi-lobed gland is situated in a protective hollow in the cranium on the midline of the ventral brain. The action of the anterior and posterior lobes is controlled by the hypothalamus from which the pituitary is separated by a small portal system of blood vessels by which communication between the two organs is achieved.

THYMUS

The thymus is made up of two yellowish lobulated parts situated either side of the trachea. The thymus is largest in the young animal where the left thymus (anterior) lies in the throat region and the right (posterior) extends down into the thoracic cavity and terminates at the anterior pericardium. As the animal matures the thymus undergoes atrophic change and the separation between the two parts increases as the thymus tissue is gradually replaced by adipose (fat) cells to the extent where the anterior thymus becomes vestigial and the posterior thymus is found only above the cardiac sac.

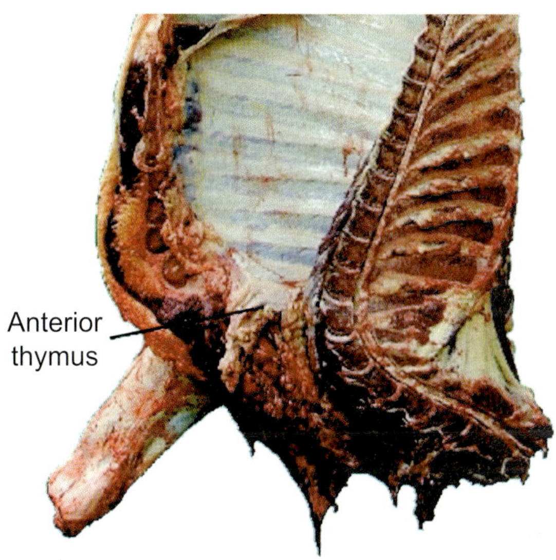

ADRENAL GLANDS

These are paired dark brown bean shaped glands approximately 3cm in length found in fat anterior to the kidneys. Each adrenal gland is composed of two differing tissues with different functions and can been seen in cross section as a dark brown cortex surrounding a lighter medulla.

PANCREAS

In addition to the exocrine function of the pancreas in the digestive process a second endocrine function is undertaken by foci of specialist cells (Islets of Langerhans) found throughout the substance of the pancreas.

Endocrine glands - summary of function

Thymus	Development and maturation of T-lymphocytes. Also sexual development.
Adrenal cortex	Produces multiple hormones (corticoids) which maintain blood volume, have an anti-inflammatory action, maintenance of blood glucose levels and fat deposition. Secretion controlled by anterior pituitary gland.
Adrenal medulla	Secretes adrenalin and noradrenalin for stimulation of cardio-respiratory system, increase in blood sugar levels and increased metabolic rate. Also raises blood pressure by vaso-constriction.
Pancreas	Insulin and glucagon work antagonistically to maintain blood sugar levels, insulin prompting conversion and storage of glucose in liver and muscles, glucagon prompting release.
Thyroid	Regulates metabolic rate through production of thyroxin prompted by hormone released by anterior pituitary in response to monitoring by the hypothalamus. Also produces calcitonin to maintain constant blood calcium levels.
Parathyroid	Secretes parathyroid hormone influencing calcium to be absorbed into bone from blood. Works antagonistically with calcitonin.
Pituitary posterior	Produces oxytocin and antidiuretic hormone (ADH). Oxytocin produced in females only, has a calming and relaxing effect during parturition and also prompts release of milk from mammary gland to the teats.
Pituitary anterior	Produces many hormones, primarily TSH (Thyroid stimulating hormone) in response to messages from the hypothalamus.

2

DISEASES OF CATTLE

INTRODUCTION

The survival of an animal depends on the symbiotic function of all the bodily systems. Disease can be considered to be an abnormality in the structure or function of these systems, and even an inability of the animal to perform as expected in relation to its peers. The traditional concept of disease is that there is a causal factor that produces recognisable macroscopic and microscopic lesions that can lead to identification of the causal factor. In this section infectious diseases are considered, including those due to viral, bacterial and fungal pathogens, be they of communicable origin (passed from one animal to another) or commensal organisms (organisms that form part of the normal microflora associated with the animal).

The role of the Meat Inspector is to determine whether the carcase or part carcase is fit for human consumption, given the macroscopic evidence of lesions presented.

Of greatest importance are zoonotic diseases, those that are naturally transmissible between vertebrate animals and man, such as anthrax and brucellosis.

ROUTES OF INFECTION

There are five routes by which infectious organisms gain entry into the host animal, these being:

- **Inhalation** – The causative agents are drawn into the body during the act of inspiration. Tuberculosis lesions usually have primary foci within the lung tissue.
- **Ingestion**- Infection and subsequent spread is achieved by entry of the infectious agent via the digestive tract, initial lesions in this tract are usually followed by transference of the infection to the liver via the hepatic portal blood circulation. Examples include endoparasites such as liver fluke and the larval stages of *Echinococcus granulosus*
- **Inoculation** – Penetration of the physical barrier to infection, provided by the skin and mucous membranes, allows entry of micro organisms, either through exposure of subcutaneous tissue to environmental contamination or by the injection of these agents that may be present on or in the object penetrating the barrier as occurs in wounds and insect bites. Examples include the tick transmitted infection of red water fever.

- **Congenital**- Vertical transmission from the dam to the offspring. If this infection occurs before the foetus has developed its own immune system (before third trimester) any infectious organism can be included in the phase where recognition of 'self' occurs so that any infection may not be countered as it is not recognised as foreign material.
- **Sexual**- Infection can be passed during copulation. Brucellosis and other forms of infectious abortion are known to be transmitted in this manner.

The initial site of microscopic or macroscopic infection is known as the primary focus. The description of condition being a peracute infection indicates rapid onset (few hours), an acute infection generally denotes one of short duration (1-2 days) as opposed to a chronic infection (1 week plus.)

IMMUNITY

Immunity can be described as non-susceptibility to a particular disease, the pathogenic effects of micro organisms, or chemical toxins. Immunity is the ability of the body to distinguish foreign material and to neutralize or eliminate it. This is achieved through the body's immune response. Foreign material is recognised by the presence of substances called antigens, which can be toxins, foreign proteins and even parts of the polysaccharide cell walls of bacteria and other tissue. The immunity of a body to infection, either exogenous (where external organisms breach the body defences) or endogenous (where natural flora become pathogenic), is dependant on the inter-reaction of three lines of defence. The first two lines of defence, the skin/mucous membranes and the cellular/humoral factors are innate and non-specific; they are a normal part of the body and react to the presence of any foreign body. The third line of defence, the acquired immune response, is specific to each individual type of invading micro organism and takes longer to mobilise. The first lines of defence form the initial immune reaction and initiate the specific response.

SKIN/ MUCOUS MEMBRANES

These form the initial defence to infection in three ways. Firstly they provide a physical barrier, which produces antimicrobial factors such as the fatty acids present in sweat, the lysosomes in mucous, and surfactant in the lungs. Secondly the mucous membranes provide a mechanical defence, wave-like movement of hair-like projections called cilia of the cells in conjunction with mucous remove foreign particles. Thirdly the presence of normal flora, known as commensal organisms, on the skin and mucous membranes compete with pathogens for space and nutrients, this competition normally involving the production of short chain fatty acids that act as microbial agents against the invading organisms.

CELLULAR FACTORS

Specialised cells (collectively known as phagocytes) free within the body systems are capable of **phagocytosis**, literally the eating of cells; these include neutrophils which primarily attack extracellular bacteria, eosinophils which attack parasites, and macrophages that attack intracellular bacteria, protozoa and viruses. The process of phagocytosis is four staged, beginning with **chemotaxis**, whereby the phagocyte is attracted to the invader by chemicals produced by the invader itself as well as the body due to the presence of the invader. The second stage is the **adhesion** of the phagocyte to the invader. This is usually accomplished by the phagocyte extending its membrane wall into a 'false limb' (pseudopodium) that reaches out and attaches to the invader. The invader is then **ingested**; the pseudopodium retracts, drawing the invader into the phagocyte, which then extends further pseudopodia around the organism trapping it in a space called a vacuole within the phagocyte. The final stage is the **killing** of the invader, this is achieved either though an oxidative burst by chemicals such as hydrogen peroxide, or through the damaging of the bacterial membrane by lysosomes present in the phagocyte. Enzymes then degrade the dead bacterium.

HUMORAL FACTORS

These assist the process of phagocytosis and are a chain of chemical reactions of serum proteins, the product of one reaction being the catalyst or initiator of the next. The products of these reactions induce chemotaxis, aid adhesion of the phagocyte, lyse (kill) organisms by breaking down the cell wall and increase the vascular permeability allowing the increased supply of phagocytes to the infected area.

ACQUIRED IMMUNE RESPONSE

This specific immune defence is acquired after exposure to infection, and forms the basis of the theory of vaccination. It relies on **antibodies**, molecules of immunoglobulins that comprise three areas, two constant that activate phagocytes and humoral responses and a third that 'keys' onto the specific antigen of the invading organism. Each microbe is therefore recognised by a specific antibody that attaches to it, attracts phagocytes and triggers the humoral factors. The acquired immune response is dependant on cells known as **lymphocytes**, of which there are two groups, characterised by their function and site of maturity. Lymphocytes are derived from stem cells that travel to areas of the body to mature. **B-cells** are antibody producing cells that are matured in the bone marrow in mammals, **T-cells** are matured and released from the thymus and are involved in cell mediated immunity and assisting the production of antibodies in B-cells.

Each B-cell produces one specific type of antibody and carries large numbers of these on its surface to act as receptors. When confronted with the infectious agent that displays the specific antigen that allows the receptors to lock, the B-cell is activated, multiplies and stimulates other plasma cells to produce copies of the antibody, producing large numbers of cloned B-cells called **affector cells**. Once the infection has been overcome, some of these B-cells remain viable as '**memory cells**' and remain present should the infectious agent be encountered in the future.

T-cells have various functions, but are primarily aimed at intracellular microbes. **Cytotoxic** T-cells recognise the antigen in virus-infected cells and kill the cell before the virus is released and also produces chemicals that create resistance to infection in neighbouring cells. **Suppressor** T-cells decrease the activity of other T and B-cells. **Helper/inducer** T-cells assist other T-cells to become cytotoxic, help B-cells produce antibodies, recognise microbial antigens in phagocytes and produce a chemical to activate the macrophage to kill the microbe.

Inflammation is a localised response to tissue damage or the presence of antigens. The local capillaries enlarge and increase permeability allowing large numbers of lymphocytes and phagocytes to enter the area, which then proceed to localise and neutralise the cause of the inflammatory response. The classic signs of inflammation are side effects of these changes and include heat, pain, swelling, redness and disturbance of function. Once the causal factor has been overcome, the result to the affected tissue can be regeneration, scarring or cell death (necrosis).

There are various forms of inflammation including those leading to the formation of fibrous tissue (fibrinous inflammation), promoting adhesion of adjacent organs or membranes (adhesive inflammation) and diphtheric inflammation, where fibrinous exudates are formed firmly attached to underlying tissue such as occurs in cases of calf diphtheria.

BACTERIA

SIZE AND STRUCTURE

Bacteria are single celled organisms classed as prokaryotic organisms, with varying shapes (morphologies) including spherical, rod shaped, comma shaped, spiral and ranging in size from approximately 0.5-6.0μm.

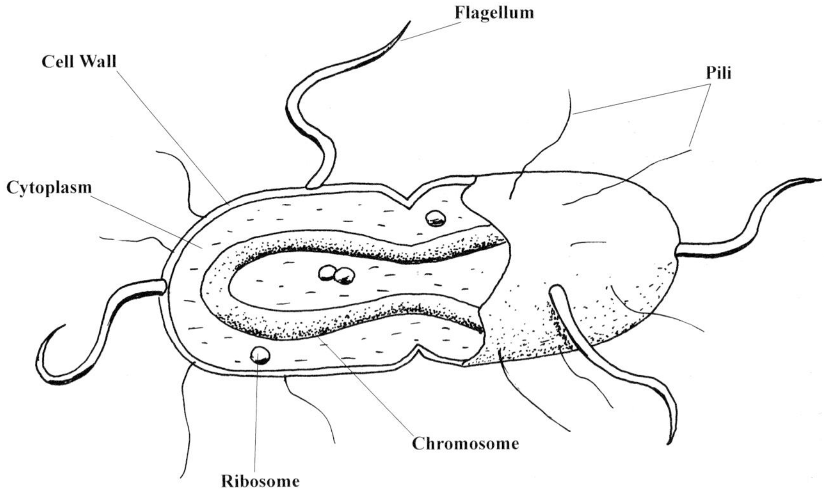

Represenative bacteria

Prokaryotic organisms (bacteria and green celled algae) are distinguished from other living organisms by containing DNA in a double stranded loop that is unenclosed by a nuclear membrane, small ribosomes (granules containing RNA), and no endoplasmic reticulum (a network of membranes within a cell involved in protein, lipid (fat) and glycogen synthesis). They are also characterised by the absence of mitochondria or other membrane enclosed organelles, and the possession of a complex protein cell wall, (with the exception of mycoplasma.)

The bacterial cell structure includes a rigid cell wall and in many bacteria a mucoid polysaccharide layer complements this. This capsule resists absorption and destruction (phagocytosis) by white blood cells and also aids adherence to tissues.

The pili (fimbrae) are hair-like in appearance, can aid attachment to host cells, are anti-phagocytic and can avoid host antibody response by rapidly altering their antigenic protein, pilin.

Flagella are much longer than pili and provide mobility for the bacterium. The bacteria can have one flagellum at one or both ends (monotrichous), many flagella at one or both ends (lopotrichous), or be 'covered with hair' (peritrichous). Mobility is achieved by clockwise or counter clockwise rotation of the flagella.

Certain bacteria have the ability to sporulate (e.g. Clostridium and Bacillus spp.), where an extremely tough protective coat surrounds concentrated bacterial DNA. The cell becomes metabolically inert and can survive dehydration, heat and most chemical agents for years, until favourable conditions for growth reactivate the bacterium.

ENERGY, NUTRITION AND GROWTH

Bacteria use three sources for their energy requirements, light (phototrophy), chemical reactions (chemotrophy) or a host cell (paratrophy).

Nutritionally bacteria can be divided into two types; autotrophs, which can synthesise nutrients from inorganic raw materials, and heterotrophs, which depend on preformed organic molecules from the environment as the source of nutrients such as some parasitic and pathogenic bacteria, that can only survive intracellularly, they possess DNA and RNA but only have a certain amount of metabolic activity.

Bacterial growth is by binary fission, where the internal contents of the bacterium halve, split and then reform into two matching bacterium, the doubling time varying from 20 minutes (*E.coli*) to 24 hours (tubercle bacilli). The process of binary fission means that one bacterium becomes two, two become four, four become eight, and eight become sixteen. Given balanced growth, where all required nutrients are available, the growth curve of bacteria follows distinct phases. After an initial lag phase, high-virulence exponential growth occurs during the log phase, followed by a stationary phase where the number of bacteria produced is equal to the number dying, which is in turn followed by the decline phase where the number dying is greater than the number produced as the available nutrients are used up.

Each bacterial species has varying requirements for optimum growth, including available nutrients, temperature, available moisture in the form of water activity (Aw), and the pH or hydrogen ion concentration of their growth medium.

Taking these factors in order, bacterial growth requires water-soluble nutrients, and high protein foods are favoured such as eggs, fish and meat. Food was historically salted to preserve it, which reduces moisture as well as preventing the osmotic diffusion of nutrients into bacterial cells.

In terms of temperature, the lower the temperature, the slower bacteria grow. Most disease causing bacteria (pathogens) cannot grow below 4°C and none can grow below 0°C, spoilage bacteria can grow at temperatures down to -5°C. As these are the only two groups of bacteria present on meat, at temperatures below -5°C all bacterial growth ceases.

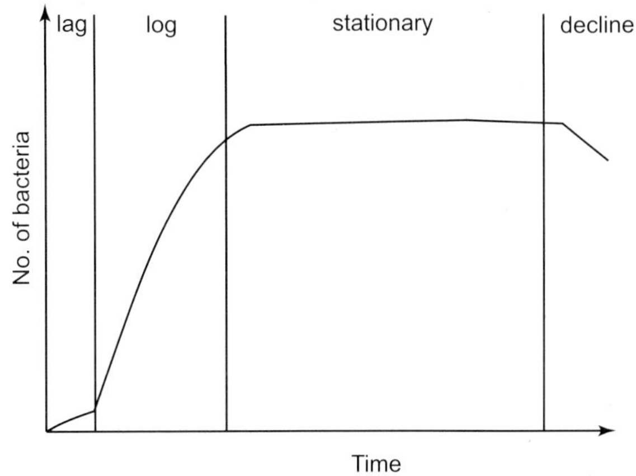

Bacterial growth curve

Each bacterial species has an optimum temperature for growth, as well as a temperature range in which they grow, it is generally accepted that there are four groups:

	Optimum	Range	
Psychrophiles	Below 20ºC	-5 to 25ºC	Includes spoilage bacteria prevalent in cold stores and refrigerators
Psychrotrophs	Above 20ºC	-5 to 40ºC	
Mesophiles	20 to 45ºC	10 to 56ºC	Includes most common pathogens such as *E.coli*, *Staphylococcus aureus* and *Campylobacter jejuni*
Thermophiles	Above 45ºC	35 to 80ºC	Important in canning

The moisture content, or available water level (Aw), is vital to the growth of bacteria. Pure water has an Aw value of 1.0. Bacteria have a preferred optimum available water value of around 0.99, however, *Staphylococcus aureus* will grow at 0.89 and some bacteria will grow as low as 0.75.

The hydrogen ion concentration, or pH, of the medium also affects bacterial growth. Water has a neutral ph of 7, pH values from 1 to 7 are decreasingly acidic (decreasing concentration of +H ions) and those from 7 to 14 are increasingly alkaline, (increasing concentration of –OH ions). Bacteria prefer mediums with a pH of around 7; most bacteria will not grow in food with a pH below 4.5.

TOXINS

Bacteria posses the ability to form toxins, chemicals that alter the characteristic of cells and tissue, both for the purpose of defence against attack, and to increase the invasive potential of the bacteria. There are two types of toxin, endotoxin and exotoxin.

Endotoxins are released into surrounding tissue only when the bacterium breaks down formed from polyliposaccharides that form part of the cell wall. Exotoxins are formed from proteins and are excreted from the cell into surrounding tissues. Bacterial Exotoxins, such as that produced by *Clostridium botulinum* (botulism) are the most potent poisons known to man.

BACTERIAL IDENTIFICATION

In general, owing to secondary infection and the fact that various bacteria can manifest themselves in similar lesions in the affected organism, identification of the infectious agent is conducted in laboratories by culturing samples.

Bacteria are classified in various ways including their shape/size, motility, resistance to antibiotics, oxygen requirements, culture media etc. One of the identifying tests conducted is Gram's staining in which the bacteria are initially stained with crystal violet, treated with iodine solution and then decolourised with alcohol. When observed under a microscope the bacterial cells either retain a deep purple colouration and are said to be Gram positive, or their complex cell wall chemical structure resists iodine and the walls are decolourised by the alcohol and are said to be Gram negative.

VIRUSES

Viruses are obligate parasites, they do not contain the biochemical mechanisms for their own replication and are unable to replicate outside of a living cell.

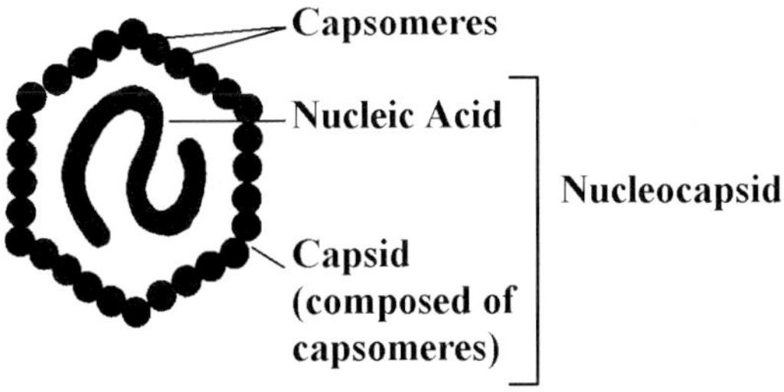

The basic viral particle (nucleocapsid) consists of linear genetic material (DNA or RNA) surrounded by a protein coat (capsid) composed of capsomeres. Some viruses are also enclosed in a membranous envelope of lipoprotein; in the case of the influenza virus this coat is formed from the host's cellular tissue and inhibits the body's auto immune response.

A virion is the complete viral particle, found extracellularly and capable of surviving in a metabolically inert form and possessing the ability to infect living cells. Virion range in size from 0.003 to 0.05 μm.

Viruses replicate by using the biochemical mechanisms of a host cell to synthesize and assemble their separate components. When attached to a host cell, only the viral nucleic acid and in some cases a few enzymes, are injected into the cell. The nucleic acid is then replicated within the cell, followed by the synthesis of the capsid.

ENVELOPED VIRUS

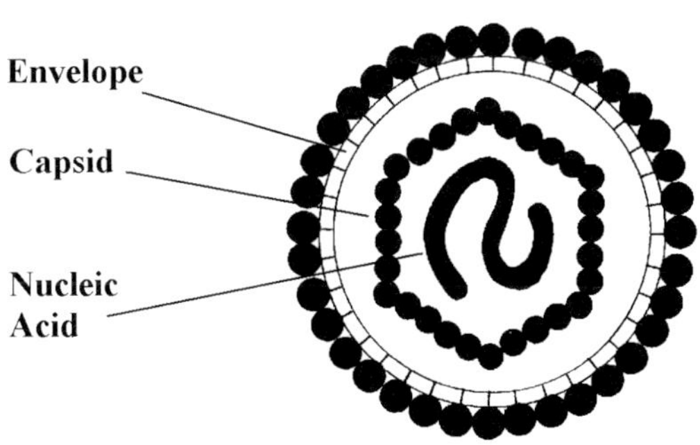

After infection by a virus, there are four possible effects on the host cell.

- Transformation of normal cells to tumour cells. Followed by division and the production of a tumour.
- Lytic infection. After viral multiplication the cell dies releasing the virus.
- Persistent Infection. After viral multiplication there is a slow release of the virus without cell death.
- Latent Infection. After viral multiplication the virus is present in the cell but not causing harm. Later emerges in lytic infection.

VIRUS TYPES

Adenovirus	Unenveloped, linear, double stranded nucleic acid.
Birnavirus	Unenveloped. (Bi=two) double stranded RNA present in two segments.
Coronavirus	Enveloped. Corona refers to the crown-like appearance of spikes on the envelope. A cytocidal, organ specific virus leading to progressive degeneration.
Herpesvirus	Enveloped. Large, double stranded, linear DNA, icosahedral capsid.
Orthomyxovirus	Enveloped. Influenza virus. Type A affects humans and animals, Types B&C affect only humans. RNA genome divided into eight RNA molecules.
Paramyxovirus	Enveloped. Infective mechanism relies on fusion of the envelope with the host cell membrane. RNA protected by helical nucleocapsid.
Parvovirus	Unenveloped. Smallest and simplest viral particle. Icosahedral capsule containing one molecule of single stranded DNA.
Picornavirus	Unenveloped. Pico-RNA literally means small RNA that is single stranded.
Pox virus	Large ovoid or brick shaped viruses, replicates in the cytoplasm of cells. First virus to be seen microscopically.

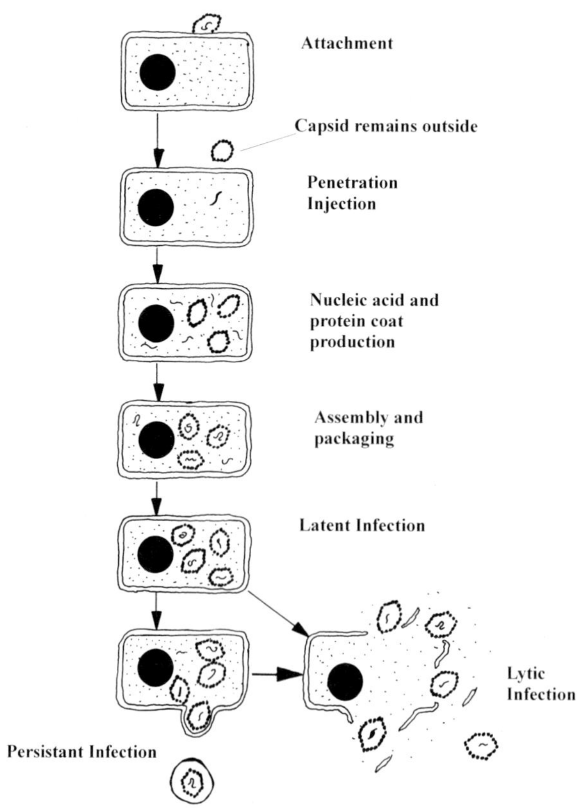

Replication cycle of a virus.

FUNGI

Fungi (yeasts, moulds etc) are eukaryotic organisms, characterised by the absence of chlorophyll, the presence of a rigid cell wall in some stages of their life cycle, and their reproduction by means of spores. Their cell size ranges between 10-30 μm, containing organelles such as mitochondria, Golgi apparatus, lysosomes and endoplasmic reticulum, and linear DNA contained in a nuclear membrane. The cells are non-motile and heterotrophic. Their reproduction is complex (asexual and sexual).

There are two major morphological forms of fungi, small round yeasts and long filaments called hyphae. Yeasts are round, unicellular and multiply by budding or by fission. Filamentous fungi form hyphae; long tubes containing protoplasm which may have cross walls, called septa, which possess a central pore allowing the through flow of protoplasm; or the hyphae may simply be multinucleate. A collection of hyphae is known as a mycelium, which may be vegetative, growing on a nutrient surface, or can extend upward as an aerial mycelium producing 'spores' (conidia) which spread very easily.

Dimorphic fungi exist in both forms. Many pathogenic fungi are dimorphic, usually with the yeast variety forming inside tissues and the filamentous (mould) form in the environment or surface.

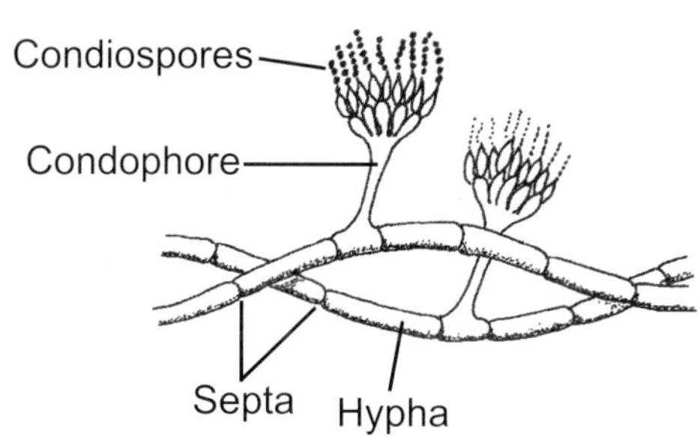

In terms of meat quality, fungi can survive on medium with a lower Aw than bacteria, and are less affected by pH. Different fungal groups produce varying physical appearances on meat, white 'whiskers' are attributable to *Mucor spp.*, green patches to *Penicillium spp.*, white spots to *Sporotrichum spp.*, and black spots to *Cladosporium spp.* They do, however, take longer to grow than bacteria, and meat spoilage is more likely to be attributable to the latter.

Various fungi produce chemicals during their growth such as antibiotics and toxins, known as mycotoxins. These secondary products of metabolism are not necessary for the growth of the fungi, but are felt to form a system to prevent competition for available space and nutrient from bacteria and other fungal species by inhibiting the growth of these other microorganisms. The antibiotics disrupt the growth of bacteria, the use of Penicillium spp. as an antibiotic is well known. Mycotoxins, when produced by fungi on foodstuffs such as grain kept in a humid environment can cause toxaemia in animals. The effects of which vary according to the level of toxin in the feedstuff, the duration of intake, and the age, sex and nutritional status of the host. Fungal toxins generally affect the liver.

PRION PROTEINS

Prion proteins are pathogenic variants of proteins that are naturally produced mainly by nerve cells. These are an infectious agent, despite not containing nucleic acid and have the same chemical composition as the normal proteins produced but have a different molecular shape and the ability to force the normal protein to alter its shape and become pathogenic. Prion proteins cause a group of diseases known as Transmissible Spongiform Encephalopathies (TSE's) that include scrapie in sheep, new variant CJD and 'Kuru' in humans and Bovine Spongiform Encephalopathy (BSE, Mad Cow Disease) in cattle.

It has long been felt that the feeding of mammalian protein in foodstuffs prompted the initial outbreak in cattle. Much research has been undertaken as to the nature and pathogenesis of prion proteins, and legal requirements for the slaughter and dressing of cattle alter in line with the emergence of new scientific advice.

When material that may contain prions is ingested (pasture contaminated by infected placental tissue from infected animals, mammalian foodstuffs etc), the prions congregate and are isolated at the Peyer's patches within the small intestine. They are then transported by lymphocytes to lymph nodes and other lymphoid material such as the tonsils, spleen and thymus. Here, replication of the prion takes place. Normal proteins are produced within cells and move via the Golgi bodies to the cell membrane. Initial encounters with rogue prion proteins forces the normal proteins to change shape and characteristic to become a prion protein, this action is the initial transmission of infection. Once altered the new rogue prion protein then infects its neighbours and so on. If the prion proteins accumulate within a cell there is also the possibility that the infection can spread during the normal protein production within the cell.

It is felt that the prion proteins may then move along nerve axons to the spinal cord and then to the brain, the exact mechanism for this movement is unclear, it may be due to the movement of vesicles within and between nerve cells or may be just a matter of spread of infection between contacting surfaces.

The replication of the prions in the brain tissue leads to the formation of non-inflammatory vacuoles and brain dysfunction, the clinical signs of which are atypical of this dysfunction; loss of motor control, paralysis and loss of control of the autonomic nervous system (dysautonomia) and finally death.

At present the accumulation of prion proteins in infected animals in certain lymphoid and nervous tissue has led to that tissue being removed from the carcase under special precautions and treated in such a way as to prevent it from entering the human and animal food chain. This material, termed Specified Risk Material currently includes the head (excluding the tongue), tonsils (including the sublingual tonsular material), thymus, salivary glands, spleen, intestines, spinal cord and brain.

DISEASES OF CATTLE

ACTINOBACILLOSIS

Synonyms	Wooden Tongue
Type	Bacterial
Aetiology	*Actinobacillus ligniersi.* Gram –ve pleomorphic rod
Pathogenesis	Considered to be a commensal organism within the bovine oropharynx, the route of infection is due to inoculation of the organism into soft tissue such as the tongue, and retropharyngeal lymph nodes. Rough herbage and foreign objects in the feed can contribute to the incidence of this condition.
Clinical Signs	An inability to feed due to the pain and reduced mobility of the tongue. A characteristic drooling of saliva is typical due to hyper salivation
Gross Lesions	Nodular lesions can be felt within the tongue tissue; these can coalesce to form hard areas hence the term 'wooden tongue'. Enlargement of the retropharyngeal, parotid and submaxillary lymph nodes can occur. When incised a non-odorous thick yellow/green pus may be found. Ingestion of infected material may introduce lesions into the digestive tract.
Judgement	The affected part should be rejected. If generalised or systemic the carcase and offal should be rejected.

ACTINOMYCOSIS

Synonyms	Lumpy jaw, Ray Fungus
Type	Bacterial
Aetiology	*Actinomyces bovis.* Gram +ve facultative anaerobes.
Pathogenesis	Considered to be a commensal organism within the buccal cavity, the route of infection is due to inoculation and entry through wounds, especially through the gum. Produces an osteomyelitis usually within the mandible. The abscessation that follows can fistulate to the surface and discharge. The term 'ray fungus' derives from the formation of a mycelium of branching filaments.

Clinical Signs	Swollen painful bones, especially the mandible and maxilla. Evidence of fistulae (scarring, depression within the skin of the cheek), flow of sticky granulatamous pus.
Gross Lesions	Honeycombed appearance of the bone due to rarefying osteomyelitis, the cavities produced normally containing thick green granulomatous pus. A quarter of cases may have lymph node involvement.
Judgement	The affected part should be rejected.

ANTHRAX

Synonyms	Wool sorters disease, Splenic fever, Charbon, Malignant pustule
Type	Bacterial
Aetiology	*Bacillus anthracis*. Large Gram +ve rod. Forms stable spores in the presence of air and remains viable in the soil for decades
Pathogenesis	Spores germinate in mucosal of throat or intestine. Rapid invasion of the bloodstream, lymphatics and spleen produces acute septicaemia. Toxin produced by the bacterium damages and kills phagocytes, increases blood vessel permeability and damages the clotting mechanism.
Clinical Signs	Death. Exudation of tarry dark blood from the natural orifices of the body. Absence of rigor mortis. Rapid decomposition of the body. Oedema Cutaneous form – Blackened raised pustule surrounded by oedema. Most common form in humans due to presence of the bacterium in open wounds.
Gross Lesions	A peracute septicaemia. Congestion throughout carcase, dark red lymph nodes and severe splenomegaly. Petechial haemorrhaging of mucous membranes, fatty change of liver and kidneys.
Other	**Zoonotic disease**. Human pulmonary form known as woolsorters disease. Cutaneous form malignant pustules. Suspect cases must not be opened for post mortem examination. *Bacillus anthracis* will sporulate in the presence of air making decontamination problematic.
Judgement	**Notifiable**. Unfit for human consumption.

BLACKLEG/ MALIGNANT OEDEMA – DIFFERING AETIOLOGY, SIMILAR PATHOGENESIS AND LESIONS

Synonyms	Malignant oedema – stable blackleg.
Type	Bacterial
Aetiology	Blackleg -*Clostridium chauvoei*. Gram –ve Malignant oedema – *Cl. septicum*. Spore forming, gas producing rods

Pathogenesis	Blackleg -Spores remain viable in the soil for years. Infection acquired through ingestion, movement through compromised digestive membrane to the body. The spores then lodge in various organs and tissues, especially muscles. Here they lie dormant until stimulated to multiply, by a reduction in oxygen usually by injury to the animal. The injury reduces blood flow to the area, thereby reducing the supply of oxygen to the tissues. In the absence of oxygen, the spores germinate and multiply. As they grow, the bacteria produce toxins which destroy surrounding tissues. The toxins are absorbed into the animal's bloodstream which makes the animal acutely sick and causes rapid death. A fatal disease of young cattle, especially those rapidly gaining weight between 6 months and 2 years of age. Produces myonecrotising toxins that kill individual muscle fibres. Malignant oedema – as above except it is more common in older cattle.
Clinical Signs	High fever, toxaemia, lameness, loss of appetite. Swellings develop in the hip, shoulder, chest and back. Starting small, hot and painful becoming swollen and gaseous. Subcutaneous emphysematous crepitation can be felt. Mortality high, usually within 12 to 48 hours due to toxaemia.
Gross Lesions	Carcases undergo rapid putrefaction. Skin over swellings can develop dry gangrene in the centre. On incision the swellings usually contain gas and discoloured serum, affected musculature contains gas and becomes black or darker than normal, and swollen. With malignant oedema gas in the musculature is normally absent.
Judgement	Unfit for human consumption

BLOAT

Type	Miscellaneous
Aetiology	Physical blockage, bacterial infection (*Streptococci bovis* a commensal organism of the digestive tract), feed type.
Pathogenesis	Two forms frothy bloat and gaseous bloat. Frothy bloat is due to surfactants in feed such as legumes forcing fermentation gas to form in frothy bubbles that cannot be eructated. Gaseous bloat can follow a rapid change in feeding leading to improper fermentation particularly of grain. It can also occur if there is physical blockage of the oesophageal orifice from the rumen.
Clinical Signs	Dyspnoea (laboured breathing) due to pressure on the diaphragm when the size of the rumen is increased. Loss of rumination, the animal literally stops 'chewing the cud'.

Gross Lesions	Grossly extended rumen. Can be a hazard of contamination, increased gas pressure can increase chances of bursting the stomachs releasing their contents.
Judgement	Fit. Animals found with bloat in the lairage should be slaughtered immediately on welfare grounds.

BOVINE MALIGNANT CATARRH

Synonyms	Malignant Catarrhal Fever
Type	Viral
Aetiology	Possibly a herpesvirus transmitted from a sub clinical infection from sheep
Pathogenesis	Viral replication in mucosal epithelium, clinical and post mortem lesions dependent on spread. Infection subdivided into peracute, head/ocular and mild forms.
Clinical Signs	Dependent on form of disease. Fever, bilateral ocular and nasal discharge, breathing difficulties, loss of appetite due to buccal and oesophageal erosion.
Gross Lesions	Head/ocular form affects eyes (cornea, eyelids). Intestinal infection-Erosive stomatitis, particularly affecting the conical papillae of the tongue, gastroenteritis with an intestinal oedema characteristic striping of the colon, vallate erosion of upper respiratory tract mucosa, lymphadenitis.
Judgement	Reject affected parts unless fever and emaciation are present warranting total rejection.

BOVINE SPONGIFORM ENCEPHALOPATHY

Synonyms	BSE, Mad Cow Disease
Type	Prion
Aetiology	Prion protein. No nucleic acid
Pathogenesis	Infection acquired via ingestion. Prions isolated initially in Peyer's patches of small intestine. Movement by lymphocytes takes the prion to predilection sites such as tonsular material, spleen and thymus. Replication of the prion in these sites is followed by propagation of the prion up nerve axons to the spinal cord and eventually the brain. Typically incubation period is from 2 to 8 years before onset of symptoms which progress over months.
Clinical Signs	Aggression, nervousness, lack of co-ordination
Gross Lesions	None. Microscopic vacuoles within brain tissue.
Judgement	Unfit for human consumption.

BOVINE VIRUS DIARRHOEA

Synonyms	BVD. Mucosal disease
Type	Viral.
Aetiology	Bovine Virus Diarrhoea Virus a Pestivirus.
Pathogenesis	Tends to affect young animals. Transmission by contact with contaminated fluids such as saliva, faeces, urine. Insect vector also a possibility
Clinical Signs	Foul smelling diarrhoea, nasal discharge, fever, recumbency.
Gross Lesions	Erosive stomatitis, rhinitis, erosion at junctions between horn/skin and mucous membranes and skin. Inflammation of the abomasum, erosion of ruminal mucosa
Judgement	Total rejection.

BRUCELLOSIS

Synonyms	Contagious abortion, Bangs Disease, Undulant fever (in humans)
Type	Bacterial
Aetiology	*Brucella abortus*. Gram –ve rod or coccobacillus
Pathogenesis	Infection acquired from intercourse with infected bulls, artificial insemination (AI) with infected semen, vaginal discharge, aborted foetuses. *Brucella abortus* can survive and grow in macrophages and has a predilection for a sugar alcohol found in high concentrations in the reproductive systems of both male and females. Abortion occurs by invasion of the placenta creating an inflammation. Death of the foetus possibly due to ingestion of infected amniotic fluid.
Clinical Signs	Abortion in cattle and premature calving, normally between the fifth and eighth month of pregnancy. Retention of the placenta is common as is post infection sterility. Hygromas at the knee joints.
Gross Lesions	Male: Orchitis, abscessation of the epididymis and testicles the latter can be replaced entirely by solid purulent material. Female: Bacteraemia and fever in aborting cow. Viscous exudates and flecks of pus between the uterus and foetal membrane.
Other	Infection in humans can be gained through contact with infected material including milk from infected cattle.
Judgement	Unfit for human consumption. **Zoonotic**.

CALF DIPHTHERIA

Synonyms	Oral necrobacillosis, necrotic stomatitis
Type	Bacterial
Aetiology	*Fusobacterium necrophorum* anaerobic gram –ve.
Pathogenesis	Commensal organism of the oropharynx.
Clinical Signs	High fever, moist cough, nasal discharge, laboured breathing, foul vegetative smelling breath.
Gross Lesions	Necrosis of the pharynx and buccal cavity. Formation of diphtheric membrane on mucosa, formed by necrotic cells and exudates adherent to underlying tissue. Aspiration can lead to septic broncho-pneumonia.
Judgement	Total rejection of carcass and offal if associated with emaciation, toxaemia or pneumonia. If localised reject affected parts.

CONTAGIOUS BOVINE PLEUROPNEUMONIA

Type	Bacterial
Aetiology	*Mycobacterium mycoides*
Pathogenesis	Easily spread by animals with sub clinical lesions and recovered animals. Occurs in acute, sub acute and chronic forms.
Clinical Signs	Coughing, laboured breathing, shallow with audible grunting. Fever, loss of appetite.
Gross Lesions	Fibrinous pleurisy with straw coloured hydrothorax. Myocardial haemorrhages, lobar pneumonia and interlobular pulmonary oedema.
Judgement	Affected parts rejected. Total rejection if associated with fever or emaciation.

CONTAGIOUS BOVINE PYELONEPHRITIS

Synonyms	Pyelonephritis.
Type	Bacterial
Aetiology	*Corynebacterium renale* Gram +ve slightly curved rod.
Pathogenesis	Predilected to the kidneys, ureters and bladder. Infection gained via the vagina during copulation or contact with contaminated material.
Clinical Signs	Urine contains blood and pus. Urination is frequent, painful and laboured.
Gross Lesions	Pale inflammation of the kidneys, medulla and renal pelvis, can also be associated with pus. Cystitis common. Renal lymph nodes enlarged. Purulent emboli within kidney can act as foci for formation of renal calculi.

Judgement	If bilateral and associated with uraemia reject carcase and offal. If no signs of systemic spread or uraemia reject affected parts.

ENTEROTOXAEMIA

Synonyms	Pulpy kidney disease, overeating disease
Type	Bacterial
Aetiology	*Clostridium perfringens* Type D
Pathogenesis	*Cl. Perfringens* is a commensal organism of the intestines. Sudden slowing of the movement of the digestive tract (for example through overeating or stock movement to lush rich pasture) allows this bacterium to multiply rapidly and it produces toxins which damage nerves and blood vessels.
Clinical Signs	Diarrhoea, bellowing, blindness, convulsions and death.
Gross Lesions	Fatty change in the liver, kidneys (hence synonym), myocardium. Pulmonary emphysema may be present as may lymphadenitis
Judgement	Total rejection of carcase and offal if toxaemia present.

ENZOOTIC BOVINE LEUKOSIS

Synonyms	Bovine viral leucosis, bovine lymphosarcomas
Type	Viral.
Aetiology	Retrovirus, genetic susceptible cattle most prone to infection.
Pathogenesis	Transmission can be through inoculation (insect vector), Maternal spread to foetus most likely. Tends to affect cattle over 1.5 years of age
Clinical Signs	Mortality high. Clinical signs dependant on organs affected.
Gross Lesions	Multiple lymphosarcomas in any organ or most commonly systemic neoplasia. Enlargement of the spleen (splenomegaly.)
Judgement	Total rejection of carcase and offal.

FOOT AND MOUTH DISEASE

Synonyms	FMD, Apthous fever.
Type	Viral. Picornavirus
Aetiology	Seven strains, A,O,C SAT(South African Territories) 1,2,3 and Asia 1
Pathogenesis	Virus extremely resistant and contagious, spread can be airborne, by fomites (inanimate objects) and through the

feeding of infected foodstuffs to other animals. Viral replication takes place in vesicles formed in the mouth and coronary bands of the feet.

Clinical Signs	Fever. Lameness. Vesicles in the mouth (tongue, gums, dental pad), interdigitally and at the coronary band of the hoof. High fever, leg shaking and 'lip smacking', a reluctance to feed.
Gross Lesions	Rupture of the vesicles leaves ulcerated mucosa covered by a flap of white epithelium. Occasionally a streaking of the heart muscle (myocardial necrosis) can be observed as longitudinal yellowish-white bands especially in calves where the condition can be fatal.
Judgement	Unfit for human consumption

FOOT ROT

Type	Bacterial
Aetiology	*Fusobacterium necrophorum.*
Pathogenesis	Damaged interdigital skin, either through penetration by foreign objects or through softening by prolonged contact with wet mud allows the organism entry.
Clinical Signs	Lameness, usually of only one foot. Pus occasionally seen. The affected foot becomes swollen and has a characteristic foul odour.
Gross Lesions	Necrotic tissue around the site of infection, pus within the wound proper.
Judgement	Reject affected part. Examine efferent lymph nodes for signs of systemic spread.

INFECTIOUS BOVINE RHINOTRACHEITIS

Synonyms	IBR, Rednose
Type	Viral
Aetiology	Bovine herpesvirus 1
Pathogenesis	Virus replicates in respiratory epithelium. Latent infection most common. Two forms, respiratory and reproductive. Respiratory -Transmission by aerosol spread. Reproductive – During copulation and parturition. Infected calves have high mortality and may develop enteric form.
Clinical Signs	Nasal discharge, rhinitis, tracheitis, conjunctivitis, hyper salivation and fever. In females can produce a vulvitis, vaginitis and consequent abortion.
Gross Lesions	Filling of nasal passages with exudates possible, can spread to trachea and lungs, petechial haemorrhaging and necrosis of mucous membranes. Bronchial and mediastinal

	lymphadenitis and bronchial pneumonia. In females pustules may appear in genital tracts. In enteric form severe gastrointestinal necrosis.
Judgement	Reject affected parts. If systemic or signs of emaciation or secondary bacterial infection (fevered, generalised lymphadenitis) reject carcase and offal.

INFECTIOUS KERATOCONJUNCTIVITIS

Synonyms	New Forest Disease, Pinkeye, Blight
Type	Bacterial
Aetiology	*Haemophilus bovis*. (*Moraxella bovis*) Gram –ve rod
Pathogenesis	Primarily insect vector spread, also damage to the cornea by grass seeds etc can promote infection.
Clinical Signs	Conjunctivitis, ocular discharge, pain and spasm of the eyelid. Reluctance to feed.
Gross Lesions	Ulceration of the cornea in chronic cases can lead to infiltration of white scar tissue and partial blindness.
Judgement	Reject affected parts

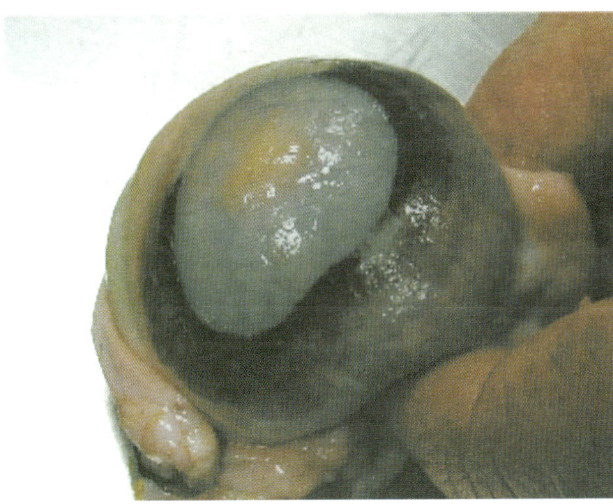

Infectious keratoconjunctivitis - corneal ulceration

JÖHNE'S DISEASE

Synonyms	Paratuberculosis
Type	Bacterial
Aetiology	*Mycobacterium paratuberculosis* Gram –ve bacterium without a cell wall.
Pathogenesis	Infection via faecal-oral route. *M.paratuberculosis* lodges in jejunal, ileal and colonic mucosa in addition to mesenteric lymph nodes. Stressors such as birth and lactation tend to

	allow the organism to reproduce to cause disease, therefore females of 2-3 years of age most commonly affected
Clinical Signs	Chronic wasting disease. Characterised by 'pipe stream diarrhoea' which is gas filled and green. Hair on coat becomes roughened. Submandibular oedema
Gross Lesions	Corrugation and thickening of the intestines. Chronic enteritis. Enlargement of mesenteric lymph nodes which become oedematous. Emaciation and oedema of the carcase.
Judgement	Carcases may be used for manufacturing purposes depending on the state of emaciation and oedema.

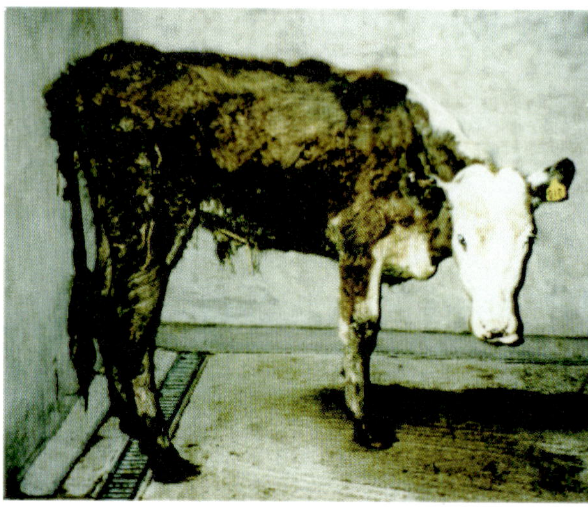

Jöhne's Disease

LEPTOSPIRIDIOSIS

Type	Bacterial
Aetiology	Leptospira species, in particular *Leptospira hardjo*. Small coiled motile bacterium.
Pathogenesis	Transmission via urine or contaminated water and inoculation of damaged skin.
Clinical Signs	Adults – Fever, abortion, mastitis, undulating fever, jaundice and anaemia
Gross Lesions	Calves – Interstitial nephritis, jaundice, acute haemolytic anaemia Adults - Ranges from anaemia, interstitial nephritis, septicaemia.
Judgement	If systemic, reject carcase and offal. If localised reject affected parts. **Zoonotic**.

LISTERIOSIS

Synonyms	Circling Disease. Listerial meningocephalitis
Type	Bacterial

Aetiology	*Listeria monocytogenes*. Gram +ve rod
Pathogenesis	Cattle with lowered resistance to disease on a high silage diet are most prone to infection. *L.monocytogenes* is an environmental bacterium multiplying in silage, soil, and grass. Thrives in aerobic conditions where the pH is 5.4 or higher.
Clinical Signs	Fever, restlessness, loss of appetite, nervous disorders including circling, leaning against objects and progressive paralysis. Mortality high in untreated cases, death can occur within 2 to 3 days from onset of symptoms but some cattle can survive for up to 2 weeks with the disease. In females with sub clinical listeriosis abortion of the foetus within the last 2 months of pregnancy can occur with possible retention of the placenta.
Gross Lesions	None in encephalitic form, but may produce focal necrosis in liver, heart, spleen and intestinal mucosa
Judgement	Reject carcase and associated offal. **Zoonotic**

PAPILLOMAS

Synonyms	Warts
Type	Viral
Aetiology	Papillomavirus
Pathogenesis	Epithelial benign tumour.
Clinical Signs	Warty growths on heads, around eyes, neck or shoulder
Gross Lesions	Initial slow growing small nodular growths turn rapidly into cauliflower like masses, either necrosis develops and they fall off or they spread further.
Judgement	Reject affected parts

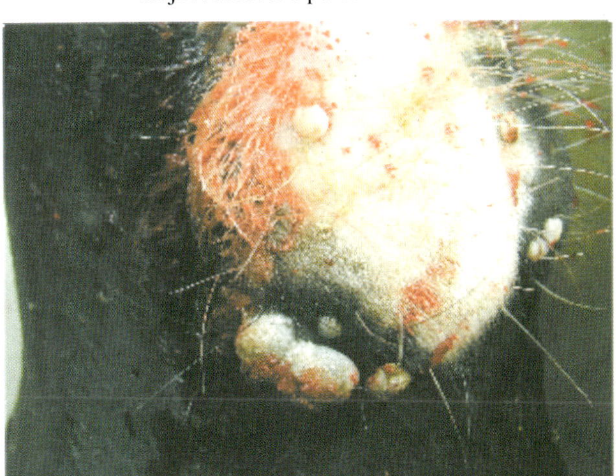

Papillomas on the ventral mandible

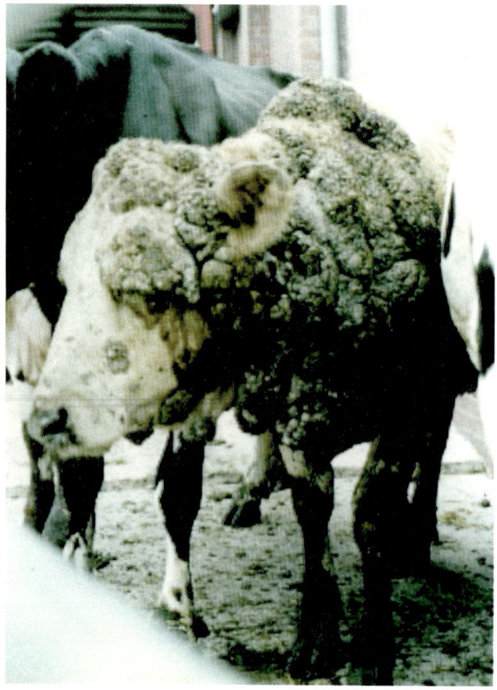

Chronic papillomatosis

RABIES

Synonyms	Hydrophobia. Lyssa
Type	Viral
Aetiology	Rhabdovirus genus Lyssavirus.
Pathogenesis	Transmission via infected saliva, usually via a bite. Very rare in cattle, most commonly infecting companion animals that have been abroad. However transmission via an infected companion animal by biting during frenzied stage is possible. Virus enters nervous tissue, spread throughout body by movement through nervous system not blood or lymphatics.
Clinical Signs	Two forms - excitation and paralytic. Excitation – Initial restlessness is followed by aggressiveness and frothy hyper salivation. Paralytic – Drooling salivation, paralysis of head and neck usually followed by paralysis and collapse of the hindquarters.
Gross Lesions	None.
Judgement	Total rejection. **Notifiable** condition in UK due to fatal outcome in infected humans.

RED WATER DISEASE

Synonyms	Bacilliary haemoglobinuria
Type	Bacterial
Aetiology	*Clostridium haemolyticum.* Gram+ve rod, spore forming.
Pathogenesis	Occurs occasionally in the UK. Produces toxins that cause intravascular haemolysis and capillary damage. Organism normally gains entry to the body either with liver fluke, or sets up in the liver where the action of liver fluke has damaged bile ducts. High mortality.
Clinical Signs	Characteristic arched back and withdrawn abdomen, shallow breathing. Haemoglobinuria (Blood in the urine), blood stained faeces.
Gross Lesions	Petechial haemorrhages throughout carcase due to capillary damage. Necrotic infarction of the liver.
Judgement	Unfit for human consumption

RINGWORM

Synonyms	Dermatophytosis
Type	Fungal
Aetiology	*Trichophyton verrucosum.* Spore forming fungi.
Pathogenesis	Germinating spores infect the hair shafts and dermis. A crusty scab forms raised from surrounding dermis. As the infection spreads outward from the primary foci the internal scab is lost leaving the characteristic ring that gives this infection its name.
Clinical Signs	Circumscribed elevated dermis, occasionally denuded of hair, can be scaly or scabby.
Gross Lesions	None. Superficial skin lesion. Secondary infection possible.
Judgement	Reject affected skin. **Zoonotic**

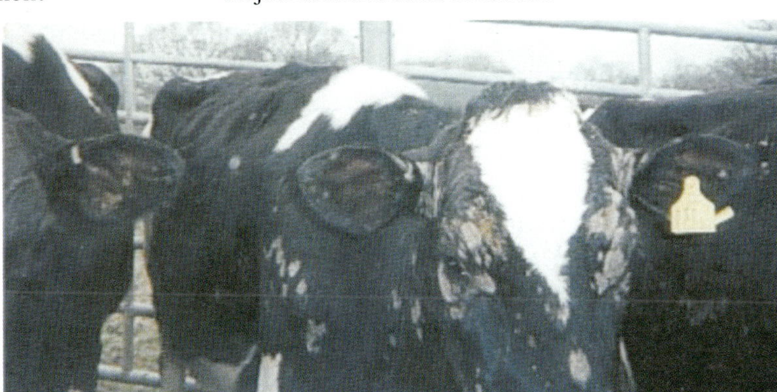

Ringworm – *Trichophyton verrucosum*

SALMONELLOSIS

Synonyms	Paratyphoid
Type	Bacterial
Aetiology	All Salmonella species including *Salmonella typhimurium. Salmonella dublin* host specific to cattle. Gram –ve short rod shaped bacteria
Pathogenesis	Three forms, chronic enteritis, acute enteritis and peracute septicaemic.
Clinical Signs	Adults – rare, tends to be associated with liver fluke infection and late to post pregnancy, can cause abortion. Calves –Tends to be peracute septicaemic form in calves up to 5 months, foul smelling diarrhoea, high fever and dehydration and rapid death (24-48 hours). Can lead to polyarthritis.
Gross Lesions	Calves- septicaemia, petechial haemorrhages in peritoneum and haemorrhagic enteritis of ileum and colon. Adults – *S.typhimurium* can produce necrotic enteritis. *S.dublin* can lead to inflammation of the abomasum. Fatty change in the liver and haemorrhagic, oedematous lymphadenitis.
Judgement	Total rejection of carcase and offal. **Zoonotic**

SHIPPING FEVER

Synonyms	Bovine Respiratory Disease. Transit Fever
Type	Bacterial syndrome, normally in conjunction with viral infection.
Aetiology	*Pasteurella multocida* and *P.haemolyticum.* Gram –ve rods
Pathogenesis	Reduced levels of immunity due to the stress of long distance transportation
Clinical Signs	Sneezing and coughing. Low grade fever.
Gross Lesions	Lobar pneumonia, fibrinous visceral pleurisy
Judgement	Reject affected parts, judge carcase on merits.

TETANUS

Synonyms	Lock Jaw
Type	Bacterial
Aetiology	*Clostridium tetani.*
Pathogenesis	Enters deep penetrating wounds, or through the umbilicus at birth. Produces neurotoxins (tetanospasmin, haemolysin) that bind to nerve membranes causing nerve excitement and continual spasmodic contraction of muscles.

Clinical Signs	Paralysis and tetanic spasms, characteristic is extension of the front legs.
Gross Lesions	No gross lesions.
Other	This disease condition highlights the need for ante mortem inspection of animals, although characteristic before death, there are no post mortem indicators.
Judgement	Total rejection.

TUBERCULOSIS

Synonyms	TB
Type	Bacterial. Gram +ve rods.
Aetiology	*Mycobacterium bovis.*
Pathogenesis	Slow developing chronic wasting disease. Various forms depending on route of infection and secondary spread. Bacterium can grow inside phagocytes; the internal spread of infection being mainly through the lymphatics, a primary focus normally develops in the afferent node for the area. Escape of bacilli into the blood circulation can lead to a generalised condition. The bacilli grow and a tubercle is formed around them, the connective tissue capsule enveloping the bacilli and macrophages and a central area of necrotic material.
Clinical Signs	As the respiratory form is the most common in cattle, coughing and progressive emaciation are the main ante mortem signs
Gross Lesions	Gross enlargement of afferent lymph nodes containing yellowish white granulation tissue. Formation of tubercles at primary foci, spread can be metastatic or through contact, respiratory TB lesions found in the lungs (apical and cardiac lobes most common) can spread to the surrounding parietal pleura forming visceral and parietal pleurisy and further tubercles which hang in grape-like clusters. Digestive TB usually follows from respiratory TB (ingestion of expectorated material) but can occur as the primary foci if infection if gained maternally. Initial sites of infection found in mesenteric lymph nodes followed by hepatic nodes then the liver and spleen proper. Miliary TB (millet seed-like) occurs when huge numbers of bacilli enter the blood stream, in this case most organs will be affected
Judgement	Reject affected parts, if systemic or generalised reject entire carcase and associated offal. **Notifiable** in UK

3

PARASITES OF CATTLE

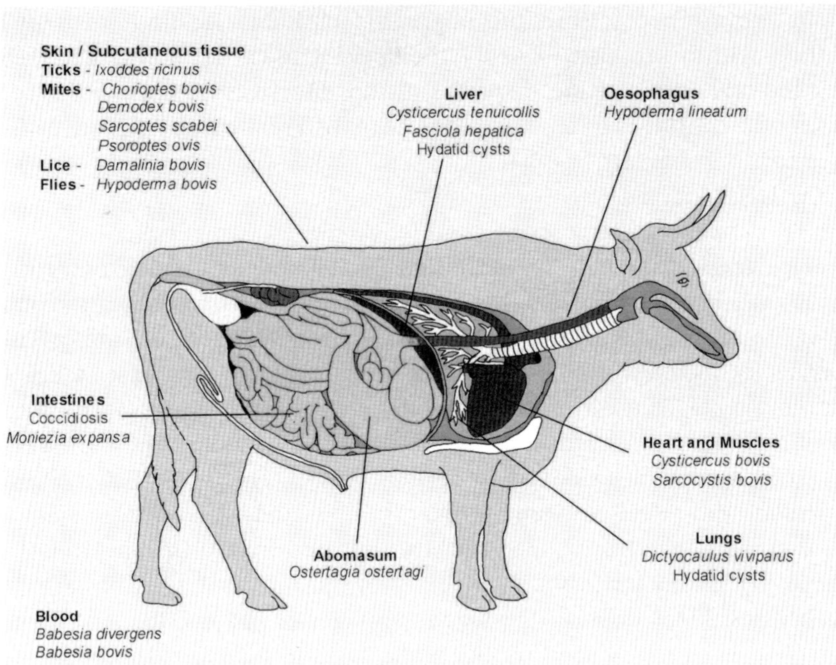

Parasites of cattle

PARASITISM

Parasites can be defined as plants or animals that live on or within another living organism at whose expense it gains some advantage whilst giving nothing in return. The host/parasite association can be complicated. The type of parasite encountered ranges from viruses (intracellular parasites) that can only reproduce in a living cell, to protozoa (single celled organisms) to intestinal worms and insects. Although they are parasitic, viruses are generally treated as a separate group, and we will only be considering parasites that are internal (endoparasites) and external (ectoparasites) that affect cattle.

Parasites may have a direct or indirect lifecycle. A direct lifecycle means that the parasite can only complete it's lifecycle by parasitizing the host.

ENDOPARASITES

HOST / PARASITE RELATIONSHIP.

The lifecycles of parasites vary, but endoparasites undergo a three-step association with the host animal. Firstly, the parasite must infect the host via the intestines, respiratory system or the skin. Secondly the individual parasite must be maintained within the host, this includes feeding, growth and migration within the host. Thirdly the species must be maintained, which means reproduction and the dispersal of the infective agents.

Each of these stages of association present different hurdles for the parasite.

INFECTION

Obviously the initial stage of parasitic development is gaining entry to the host animal. The parasite has to survive in some form in the atmosphere, whilst remaining available to enter the host. The lifecycle of most endoparasites includes a hibernation stage, for example as a cyst or egg (the infective agent) where the immature parasite lies dormant until suitable conditions trigger the release of the agent. The availability of the infective agent to host entry is achieved in various ways; some stages of a lifecycle may include the infective agent existing in a secondary or intermediate host such as worms, beetles or ants that are ingested by the primary host. The single overriding factor in the availability of the infective agent to host entry is mathematical. Infection of the host is a matter of chance; the vast numbers of infective agents produced by the adult parasite increases the odds.

Cattle are important in the respect that they not only act as the final host to parasites; they also act as intermediate host in the lifecycle of a human tapeworm, human infection occurring when a viable cyst is ingested in undercooked beef.

INDIVIDUAL MAINTENANCE

Once the agent has entered the host's body, by whatever means, it has to be able to migrate to its preferred site of habitation (predilection site), where it can mature. This can involve migration through body tissue or at the very least passage through the digestive system. Some parasites use the digestive process to activate the infective agent, others produce secretions to neutralise the effects of the gastric juices. The migration and settling of the immature parasite will also prompt the host animal's immune response to a foreign agent, this is overcome by some parasites by protective secretions, and actively encouraged by others as part of their lifecycle, using the immune response to isolate them and encase them in fibrous material where they form cysts.

PARASITE MAINTENANCE

On reaching the site where they mature, the parasite takes nutrients from the host to mature. A successful parasite can be considered one that infects, lives, reproduces and infects other hosts without killing the primary host.

SPECIES MAINTENANCE

The role of any organism, from bacterium to human, is propagation of the species. Eggs are passed by mature parasites in the faeces, and become infective agents, and the cystic stages of other parasites gain entry into the host through ingestion.

CYSTICERCUS BOVIS

Cysticercus bovis is the name given to the cysts formed by the embryos of the **tapeworm of MAN,** *Taenia saginata,* in the muscles of cattle, the intermediate host. The cysts are greyish-white, round and up to 1cm in diameter. The fact that this is a human tapeworm increases its significance in meat inspection, and most countries inspection procedures give specific actions to be taken on discovering the cysts in the carcase.

In humans the tapeworm inhabits the small intestine, the adult growing to between 5 and 15 metres in length. The worm consists of a head with four suckers, a neck and a chain of segments (proglottids) forming the stroblia. Each proglottid is budded from the neck and becomes mature as it moves down the chain. When mature the hermaphroditic proglottids produce approximately 250,000 eggs (embryophores) which either pass out in the faeces through a genital pore in the proglottid, or are passed out in a shed proglottid which then disintegrates shedding the eggs. Each egg contains a single embryo (onchosphere.)

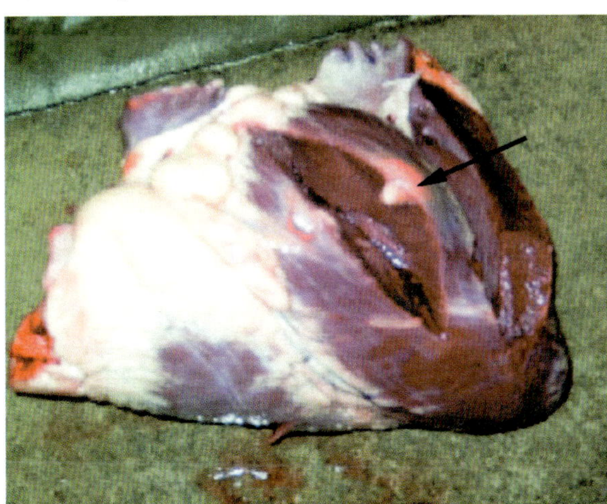

A *C.bovis* cyst in a heart. Note the way the cyst protrudes from the cut surface.

Lifecycle of the human tapeworm *Taenia saginata*

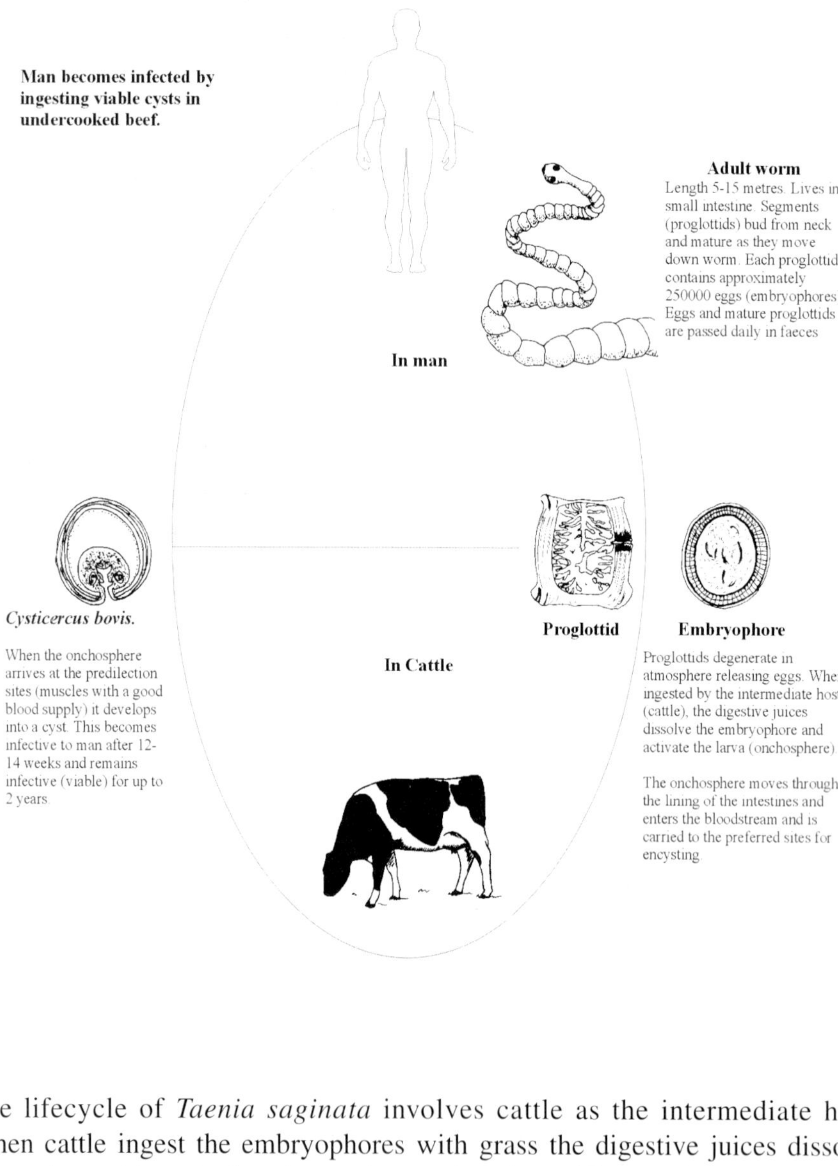

The lifecycle of *Taenia saginata* involves cattle as the intermediate host. When cattle ingest the embryophores with grass the digestive juices dissolve the embryophores and activate the onchosphere. The onchosphere travels via the bloodstream to its predilection sites (muscle with a good blood supply such as the heart, masseter, tongue, diaphragm etc.) where it forms a fluid filled cyst, a cysticercus. When viable, the cyst is transparent. The cyst can become enclosed (caseous) by the action of the bodies' immune system; after a period of time the cyst can become completely calcified at which point it is inert. Man ingesting the viable cyst in undercooked beef completes the lifecycle.

At the inspection point certain legislative procedures are followed to specifically examine for *Cysticercus bovis*, including the incision of the masseter and pterygoid muscles of the head, palpation of the tongue and skirt and visual examination and incision of the heart. If cysts are found throughout the carcase, both the carcase and offal are rejected as unfit for human consumption. If one viable or caseous cyst is found the affected part is rejected and the remainder of the carcase is refrigerated at either -7°C for 21 days or -10°C for 14 days before being passed as fit for human consumption.

FASCIOLIASIS

Fascioliasis is the term given to the change of state in cattle due to the actions of the liver fluke, a parasitic trematode called *Fasciola hepatica*.

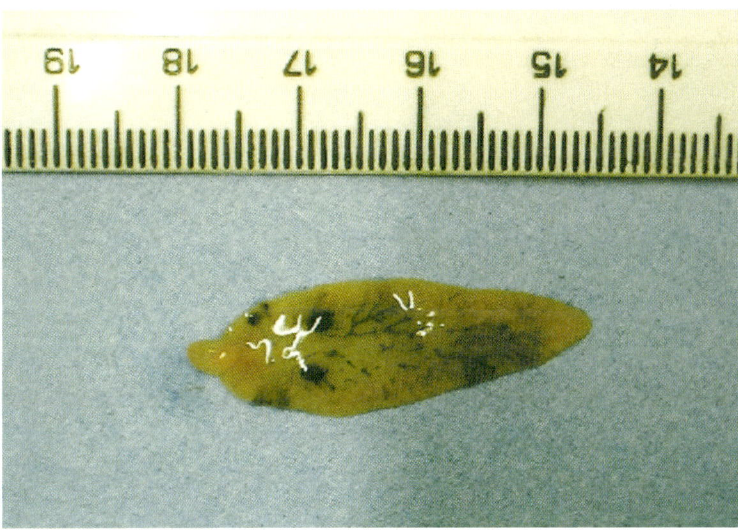

Adult *Fasciola hepatica*

Fasciola hepatica has a complicated life cycle, (see diagram for summary,) involving the mud snail *Lymnaea truncatula*. Cattle pastured in damp fields between May to June and August to October are particularly susceptible as this is when the temperature, conditions, and snail population favour the parasite.

Fascioliasis may be acute, sub- acute or chronic. Cattle tend to rarely suffer from acute fascioliasis as they do not eat grass down close to the ground water level (unlike sheep); they therefore tend not to routinely ingest the infective metacercaria that encyst at the water level of the grass.

Acute fascioliasis occurs 2-6 weeks after the beast ingests huge numbers of metacercaria (2000+), and their subsequent migration through the liver causes massive haemorrhage and damage to the liver. Acute fascioliasis can cause sudden deaths in a herd during autumn and early winter.

Sub acute fascioliasis occurs, again, in autumn / early winter, when metacercaria are ingested over a longer period and the immature fluke are at varying stages of development, some have reached the bile ducts and are causing inflammation, others are still migrating through the liver substance causing haemorrhages.

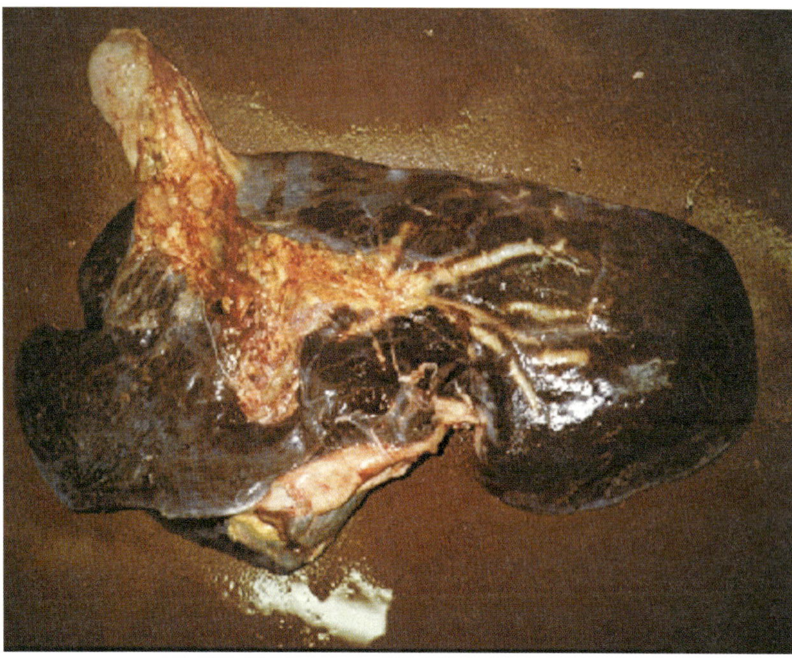

Distension of the bile ducts associated with chronic fascioliasis.

Chronic fascioliasis occurs normally in early spring; 4-5 months after 200-500 metacercaria are ingested. This form is the most common. The cattle suffer loss of condition, emaciation due to lack of appetite and the effect of the fluke on the metabolism of food. Each fluke can cause the leakage of 0.5ml of blood into the bile ducts per day, as well as plasma proteins. The liver is fibrous and the bile ducts inflamed (cholangitis.)

Submandibular oedema (bottle jaw) is a common clinical finding in chronic fluke infection.

Livers affected by adult fluke, or the migrations of immature fluke are rejected as unfit for human consumption.

Life cycle of the liver fluke *Fasciola hepatica.*

Minimum 17-18 weeks at optimum temperatures.

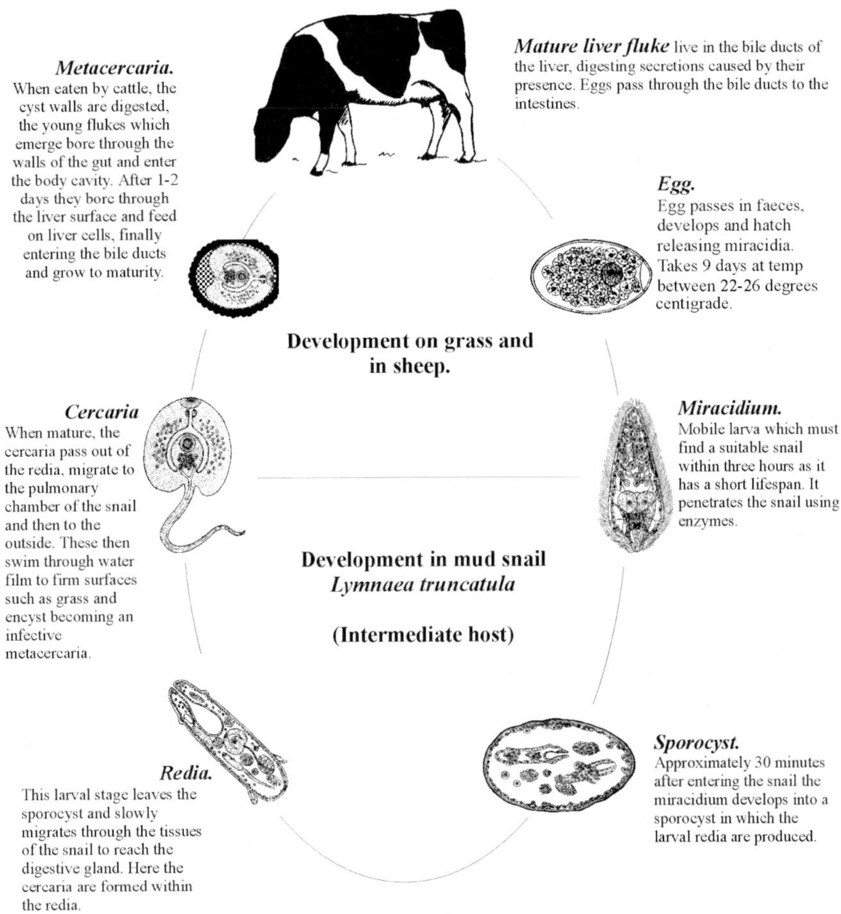

The damage caused by the presence of fluke can also lead to conditions such as Black disease, where spores of the bacterium *Clostridium novyi* germinate and multiply in the fibrotic liver as the localised blood supply and therefore the oxygen presence reduces, which could warrant the rejection of the entire carcass as well as reducing the yield of that carcass

HYDATIDOSIS

Hydatidosis is the condition where fluid filled cysts of the intermediate stage of the tapeworm of the dog *Echinococcus granulosus* are found in the internal organs, normally the liver or lungs.

Echinococcus granulosus is found in the canine intestine and is approximately 6mm in length. It consists of a head or scolex and three or four segments. The eggs (embryophores) contain one embryo (onchosphere), which has six oral hooks, and are passed in the faeces at a rate of one per week. The onchosphere can remain viable outside the host on the ground for up to two years.

When the intermediate host ingests the embryophore, the onchosphere penetrates the gut wall and travels in the blood to the liver, or in the lymphatic system to the lungs. Occasionally onchospheres escape into the general circulation and cysts are formed elsewhere in the body.

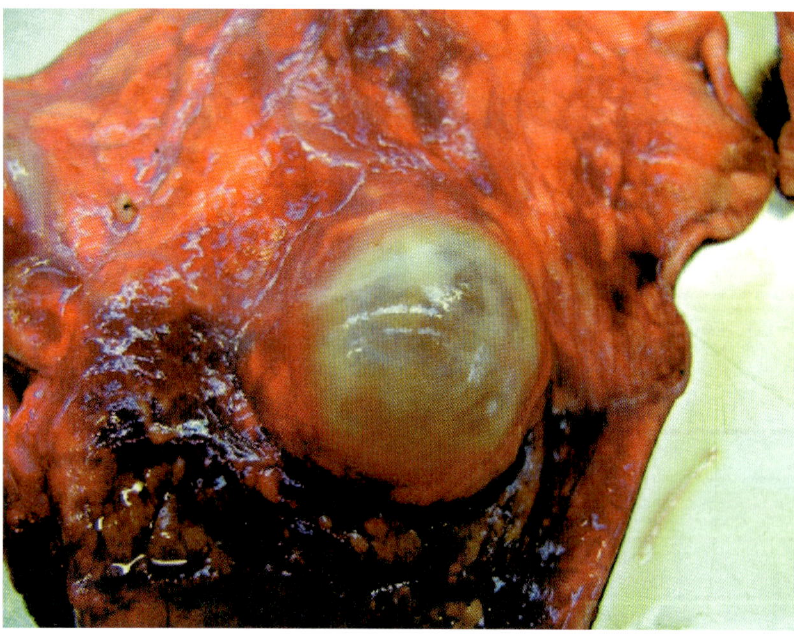

A hydatid cyst in bovine lung tissue

Humans can also be intermediate hosts, when onchospheres are ingested accidentally from the coats of dogs or transferred by dogs when licking humans, or from eating vegetables or other foodstuffs contaminated by dog faeces.

The cysts (hydatid) are slow growing, reaching maturity in 6-12 months. In the liver the cysts can reach a diameter of 20cm. Each cyst is fluid filled and contains a large number of scolices, which occasionally become detached from the cyst wall and float freely in the fluid, giving rise to the term 'hydatid sand.'

The lifecycle is completed when a dog ingests the viable cysts.

Offal containing hydatid cysts are rejected as unfit for human consumption.

LUNGWORM

The main lungworm of importance in cattle is *Dictyocaulus viviparus*, a thread-like slender worm up to 8 cm in length that colonize the trachea and bronchi of the lungs.

Dictyocaulus viviparus infection produces a condition known as husk or hoose. It causes chronic coughing and unthriftyness and severe cases can lead to lung oedema and emphysema. In the live animal the signs of lungworm infestation vary with the numbers of parasites involved. Mildly affected animals cough occasionally, especially during exercise. Those with a medium infestation cough at rest and have an increased breathing rate. Severely affected animals have a severely increased breathing rate and give the appearance of struggling for breath. Small calves are often most badly affected and death rates amongst these can be high.

The adult worms live in the bronchi where they lay eggs. These hatch and the larvae travel up the trachea to the pharynx, where they are swallowed and pass out with the faeces. They then move to grass where they are ingested by other hosts. The larvae then penetrate the intestinal wall, pass to the mesenteric lymph nodes where they moult. The larvae travel through the lymph ducts and blood capillaries to the lungs where they break into the alveoli (the blind ends of the bronchioles.) The final moult occurs in the bronchioles from where they move into the bronchi and mature. An incision into the lung tissue, cutting through the bronchi reveals thread like worms in severe infestation.

Lungs infected with *Dictyocaulus viviparus* are rejected as unfit for consumption. Secondary infection by bacteria may warrant rejection of the carcase if the infection becomes systemic

SARCOCYSTS

Sarcocysts are a sub-group of single celled parasitic organisms called protozoa. They have a two-host lifecycle, the main species found in cattle, *Sarcocystis fusiformis* being transmitted in the faeces of dogs and foxes. Studies have shown that approximately 35% of sheepdogs and up to 75% of hunting dogs are affected, possibly due to being fed undercooked beef. Another species *Sarcocystis hominis* is transmitted in human faeces.

Sarcocysts are the cystic stage of the lifecycle, which can be discerned with the naked eye, and are found embedded in muscle. These cysts are known as Meischer's tubes, roughly oval, up to 10 mm in length and are an off white/green colour. The earlier stage, sporocysts, develop in and destroy cells in the lining of blood vessels, and can cause anorexia, fever, anaemia, a reluctance of the animal to move, and abortions.

The judgement depends on the severity of the infection, localised areas can be trimmed and rejected, if the infestation is generalised the entire carcase and associated offal is rejected as unfit for human consumption.

COCCIDIOSIS

Coccidiosis is a disease condition caused by the actions of the coccidian protozoan parasite *Eimeria bovis*.

Protozoa are single-celled organisms that, unlike bacteria, possess a nucleus and other organelles that enable them to lead an independent existence. Protozoa are mobile organisms, using methods of propulsion such as flagella, cilia and undulating membranes. They feed by enveloping particles and digesting them, followed by the extrusion of waste material from the cell.

Eimeria bovis is an intercellular parasite of the cells that line the internal surface of the intestines (epithelial cells) and lacteal channels and cause lesions by destroying the cells as part of their lifecycle. The severity of the disease is dependant on the number of infective agents ingested, but an infected individual can pass several hundred million of these agents in faeces during the course of the disease.

Lifecycle. (See also Diagram overleaf). There are three basic stages in the lifecycle of *Eimeria* species, **Sporulation** occurring outside the host, **infection** and **Shizogony**, and **Gametogony** (oocyst formation).

Sporulation – eggs, or oocysts (resistant shell surrounding protoplasm and a nucleus) are passed in the faeces. Under optimum conditions, within 2-4 days the nucleus divides to produce four sporoblasts, each containing two sporozoites (the infective agent). The sporoblasts secrete a covering wall to form sporocysts. This make up, four sporocysts containing eight sporozoites, is indicative of *Eimeria* species and is used as a diagnostic method.

Infection and Shizogony. (Asexual reproduction.) – When ingested by the host, either through eating vector organisms such as earthworms that have ingested oocyst, or by ingestion of oocysts during feeding, the sporocysts are liberated from the oocyst by the digestive processes of the host animal. The sporozoites are activated by the presence of bile and trypsin in the small intestine and leave the sporocyst, and are now known as trophozoites. The trophozoites enter epithelial cells in the intestine and forms schizonts, in which division of the trophozoites nucleus forms merozoites. When the shizont containing merozoites is mature, the shizont and host cell rupture, allowing the merozoites to enter other epithelial cells where the process is repeated.

Gametogony (Sexual reproduction.)- Eventually the merozoites enter a host cell and develop into either a male form (microgametocyte) containing microgametes (small, actively mobile, flagellated organisms, similar in function to sperm), or develop into the female from, the macrogametocyte, which are single celled and expand to fill the host cell. When the microgametocyte is mature, it ruptures, together with the host cell and releases the microgametes. One microgamete then enters the host cell containing the macrogametocyte, penetrates the latter, and fusion of the two nuclei takes place. A cysts wall then develops forming a zygote that is later released as an unsporulated oocyst in the faeces when the host cell ruptures.

LIFECYCLE OF *EIMERIA SPP.*

Phase 1. Sporulation. Egg (oocyst) passed in faeces. Nucleus divides twice forming four sporoblasts. The content of each sporoblast divides into two, forming 8 sporozoites (the infective agent) per egg. The sporoblast secretes a wall to become a sporocyst. This stage occurs outside the host.

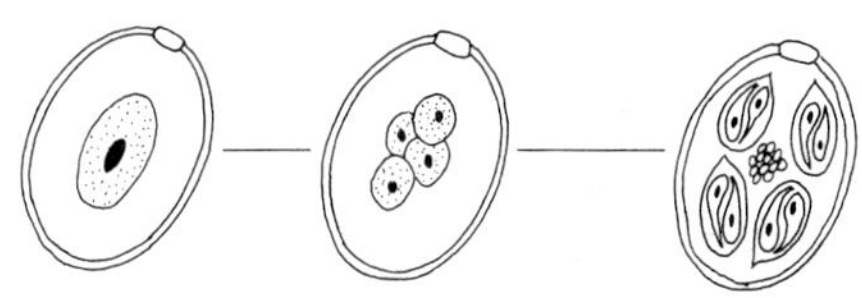

Phase 2. Infection and Shizogony. (Asexual reproduction.) When the sporulated oocyst is ingested the digestive processes of the host free the 4 sporocysts. Bile and trypsin in the intestines activate the 8 sporozoites, which leave the sporocysts. The sporozoites, now known as trophozoites, enter host cells and develop into a shizont containing merozoites. When the schizont is mature, it and the host cell rupture and the merozoites are released to invade neighbour cells. This process is repeated, the number of repetitions being species dependant.

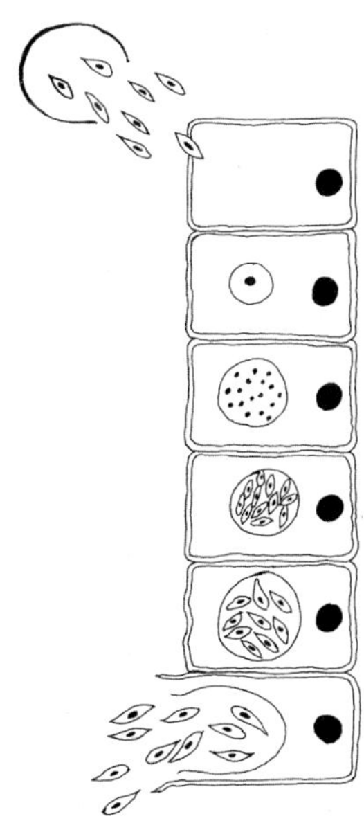

Phase 3. Gametogony. (Sexual Reproduction) Eventually, merozoites entering host cells develop into either male microgametocytes or female macro-gametocytes. The males undergo division to form mobile, flagellated microgametes within the micro-gametocyte. The female macro-gametocyte enlarges to fill the host cell. When the male host cell ruptures, the microgametes are freed, when one enters the macrogametocyte the male and female nucleus combine. A cyst wall is formed creating an oocyst, which is passed in the faeces.

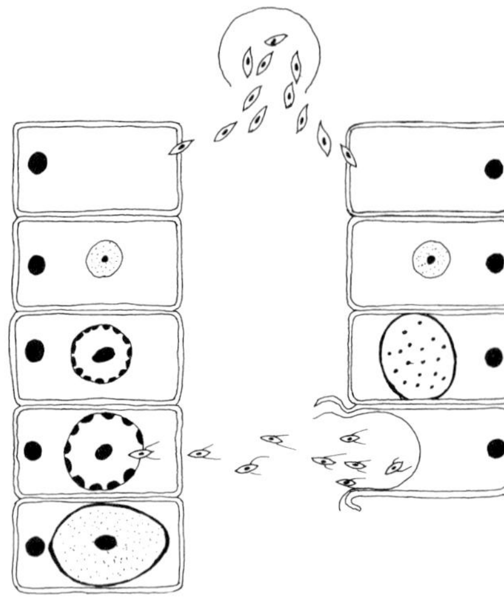

AFFECTS ON THE HOST

Eimeria species are host-specific, which is to say that a species that affects cattle will not infect sheep and vice versa. Cattle, like other animals affected by species of Eimeria can develop certain immunity to infection from exposure to previous infections, however this acquired immunity is again species specific, only relevant to the species of Eimeria encountered. The susceptibility to infection is also increased by the presence of other disease conditions that may lower the immune response. Calves and yearlings are most prone to infection.

BABESIOSIS

Also known as haemosporidiosis, piroplasmosis and Red Water Fever.

Babesia bovis and *Babesia divergens* are intraerythrocitic protozoal parasites transmitted by the tick *Ixodes ricinus*.

The organism lays singly or in pairs in cattle red blood cells and eventually divides by binary fission and ruptures the cell, releasing the organism to infect other red blood cells. When infected blood is ingested by a tick the organisms undergo their sexual phase in the gut of the tick followed by shchizogony which in turn produces motile vermicules. These vermicules multiply in the tissues of the tick and eventually invade its eggs to continue reproduction in the larvae when it hatches. The vermicules eventually migrate to the salivary areas of the larvae and form the infective sporozoites which are injected into the cattle host when the larvae feed.

The clinical signs of babesiosis are due to the wholesale destruction of the erythrocytes and release of haemoglobin and include jaundice, anaemia, splenomegaly and haemoglobinuria (the presence of free haemoglobin in the urine – 'red water').

The judgement in these cases is dependent on the condition of the animal and carcase such as rejection for icterus and anaemia.

CYSTICERCUS TENUICOLLIS

Although this parasite is included it is uncommon in cattle, however it may be responsible for parasitic hepatitis.

Cysticercus tenuicollis is the name given to the fluid filled cysts formed by the embryo of the tapeworm of the dog called *Taenia hydatigena*. The adult tapeworm can be up to 5 metres in length made up of a head and segments and lives in the intestine of the host animal. Eggs and segments are passed in the faeces of the host.

When ingested by the cattle (the intermediate host) the intestinal secretions digest the outer membrane (the embryophore) of the egg and activate the embryo (onchosphere). Using its hooks the onchosphere tears through the lining of the intestine to reach the bloodstream whereby it is carried to the liver. The onchospheres migrate through the liver substance for about 4 weeks before emerging at the surface and entering the abdominal cavity. The embryos attach to the internal surface of the abdomen, lose their hooks and develop into a large fluid filled sac containing a single head or scolex.

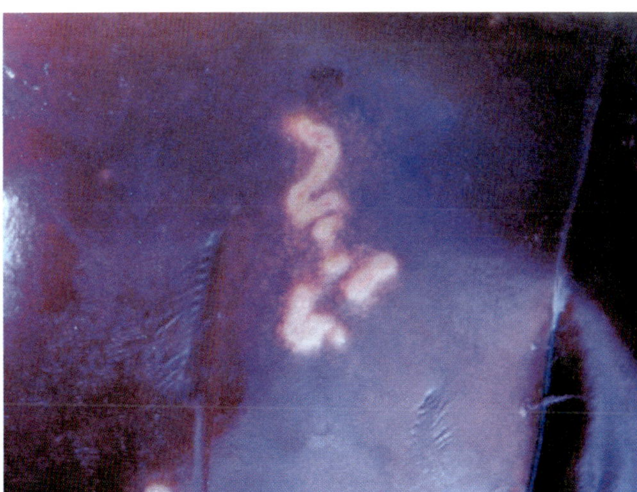

Typical 'serpentine tracts', scar tissue left by migrating larvae

The life cycle is completed when a dog eats the viable cyst.

At post mortem inspection, the migration of the onchospheres through the liver substance is indicated by 'serpentine tracks' throughout the liver. If these are evident the liver is rejected as unfit for human consumption.

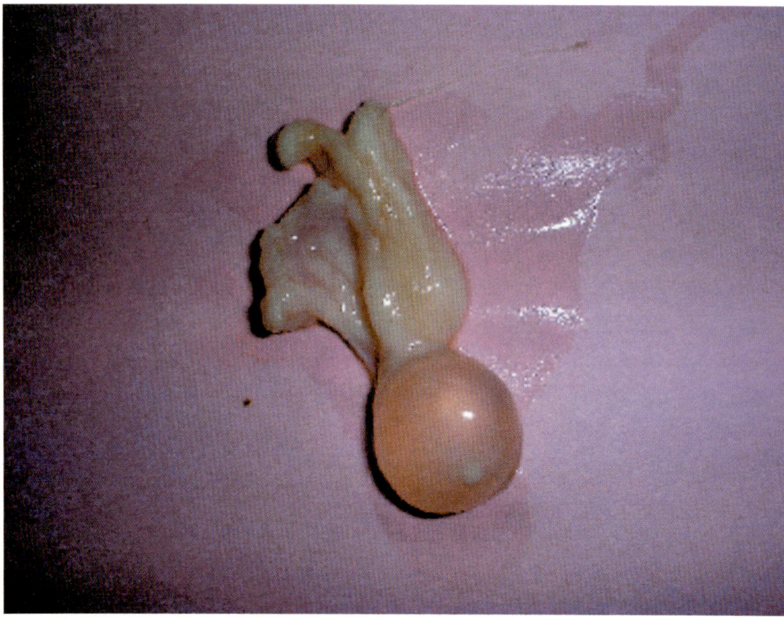

The single scolex is clearly visible in this cyst

In general, possibly due to the level that the infective agent encysts in pasture, and to a certain amount of genetic immunity or other factors, tenuicollis cysts tend to be rare in cattle.

OSTERTAGIOSIS

Ostertagiosis, also known as parasitic gastritis is caused by the nematode *Ostertagia ostertagi*, a reddish brown worm, up to 1cm in length as an adult that affects the abomasum in cattle. *O. ostertagi* is part of the same superfamily of nematodes as *Dictyocaulus viviparus* that causes parasitic bronchitis.

Ostertagia ostertagi has a direct lifecycle. Eggs are passed in the faeces and mature in the pat, the third stage larvae migrate to the surrounding soil and grass within two weeks under optimum conditions of temperature and moisture. Infection is then acquired by ingestion. The larvae then enters the gastric glands of the abomasum and moults a further two times before emerging and maturing on the surface of the abomasum. This double moult can occur approximately three weeks after infection but can also be arrested for up to 6 months depending on the time of year and environmental conditions that prevail on infection.

Clinical ostertagiosis is usually manifested in two forms, one that affects calves during their first year on pasture and a more serious form in yearlings due to the eruption of immature worms that have had arrested development from the previous year.

The effects of a heavy infestation can be severe. The kidnap and destruction of large numbers of gastric glands and the pressure the growing larvae exerts on neighbouring acid producing cells dramatically disrupts the ability of the abomasum to produce gastric juice. This cell to cell disruption can lead to an abnormal increase in the formation of new cells (hyperplasia) of the gastric surface, oedema and excess blood (hyperaemia) in the abomasal folds and eventually sloughing off of an almost diphtheric mucous membrane. The emergence of the immature worms is accompanied by the formation of characteristic nodules on surface of the mucosa.

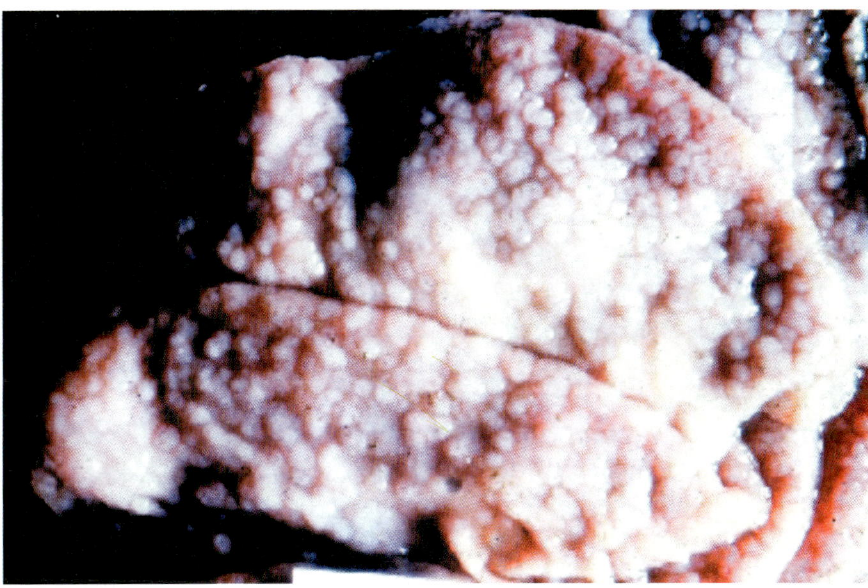

Nodules with central depression on the internal surface of the abomasum, characteristic of ostertagiosis

In conjunction with the presence of adult worms on the surface of the abomasum the affects on the animal are those initially associated with failure of the digestive system including an inability to deaminate proteins due to the loss of acidity of the gastric juice, this loss also inhibiting the antimicrobial properties of the abomasum. The damage to the epithelium of the abomasum also permits larger molecules to move directly from the abomasum into the circulation.

In the live animal a slight infection will reduce the expected weight gains, in heavy infestations there is a reluctance to eat, diarrhoea, submandibular oedema and marked weight loss.

WARBLES

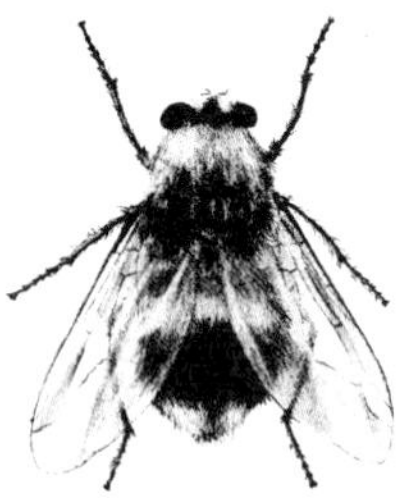

Warble flies, also known as gad flies, principally *Hypoderma bovis* (pictured left) and *Hypoderma lineatum* are active during the summer months. *Hypoderma bovis* resembles a bee in colour and will follow cattle for up to 5 Km. Cattle are irritated by their approach and tend to avoid the fly, giving rise to the term 'gadding'. The fly lays eggs on the hair shafts (singly on the lower body with *H. bovis* and in rows of 6 or more on the legs above the hocks with *H. lineatum*) which hatch in 3-7 days, the initial larval form being around 1mm in length. Upon hatching the larvae burrow through the skin using proteolytic enzymes and migrate to their over wintering site (the sub mucosal layer of the oesophagus in the case of *H. lineatum* and the epidural fat of the back (lumbar) region in the case of *H. bovis),* feeding on their way. At these sites, normally reached by late autumn the initial larva moult to the second stage.

In early spring the second stage larva of *H.bovis* migrate to under the skin of the back where they moult to the final stage. These larvae can be felt under the skin where they perforate the hide to breathe. After approximately 5 weeks the 25mm long larvae burrow through the hide to emerge and fall to the ground where they pupate for a further 5 weeks before the adult emerges.

The final larval stage under the skin creates an effect known as 'butchers jelly', where their presence causes surrounding tissues to become greenish and jelly-like, this area is trimmed and rejected. Occasionally the larvae over-wintering in the spinal canal die and release proteolysin enzyme, which can cause paralysis.

Warble fly infestation is a Notifiable Condition in the United Kingdom.

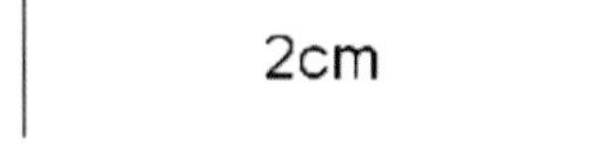

Warble final stage larvae

TICKS

Ticks are blood sucking arachnid parasites with four pairs of legs. These are important parasites in terms of inspection not only due to the blood loss a major infestation can cause, but because they represent a transport vector for various diseases including Lyme's Disease and Babesiosis, as well as biting humans.

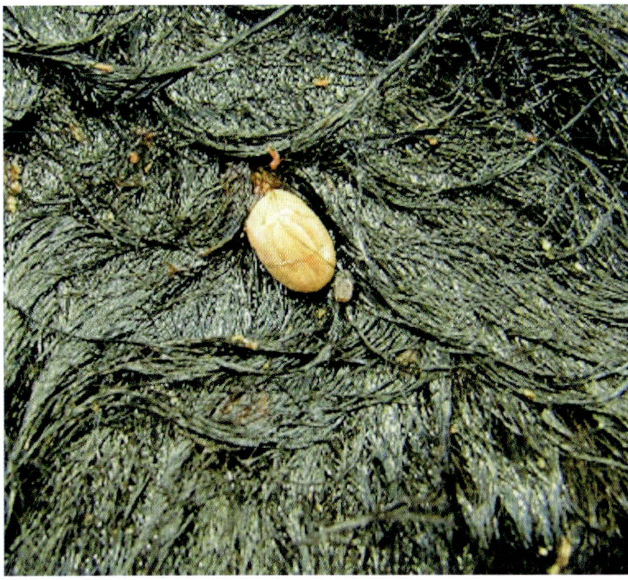

Although there are various types of tick in this country, the genera *Ixodes ricinus* is the most important in terms of disease. *Ixodes ricinus* is a hard tick, known as a three-host tick, a temporary parasite, each stage of the development taking place on a different host. The females are larger than the males and can reach a length of 1cm. Each tick feeds only three times during its three-year lifespan, once as a larva, once as a nymph and once as an adult. After mating on the host the female engorges with blood over a period of approximately a fortnight, falls from the host and lays thousands of eggs before dying. The larvae hatch and feed from a second host before again falling to the ground and moulting to the nymphal stage which feeds from a further host before dropping off and becoming an adult. In total a tick will only parasitize hosts and feed for three to four weeks during its lifespan.

Generally considered to be a parasite associated with rough herbage, infestation occurs seasonally in the British Isles, where each stage of the tick travels to the tips of plants and awaits passing animals, usually in two periods March-June and August-November where the relative humidity and temperature favours the survival of the tick.

The affects of tick infestation can be anaemia in heavy infestations but is mostly limited to secondary infection of the bite wounds by bacteria such as *Staphylococcus aureus*, also blowfly myiasis (attraction to the wounds caused by the biting), but most predominant is the transfer of rickettsial infection such as red water fever, and spirochete infection such as Lyme's disease.

MITES

Mites are insects from the same class as spiders and ticks. There are both parasitic and non-parasitic forms with the parasitic forms being further subdivided into burrowing and non-burrowing mites. There are four main parasitic species of mite encountered on cattle in the UK, all of which collectively cause a condition known as mange, these being; *Sarcoptes scabei*, *Demodex bovis*, *Chorioptes bovis* and *Psoroptes ovis*. These cause the respective conditions of sarcoptic mange, demodectic mange, chorioptic mange and psoroptic mange the latter of which is known as sheep scab in ovines.

The effect of these ectoparasites on the live animal is extremely debilitating, intense itching (pruritus) of the hide leads to rubbing, secondary infections, wounds and a preoccupation that overcomes the desire to eat. Economically infections reduce milk yield, hide value, the animals feed conversion rate and can lower the animals' resistance to other diseases.

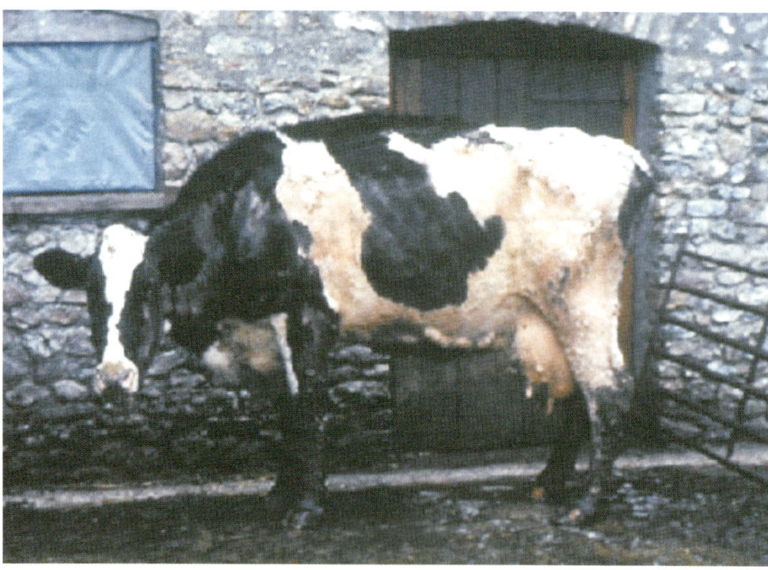

Chronic mange in a milk cow. Note areas of denuded hide

BURROWING MITES

Sarcoptes scabei is a roundish mite approximately 0.5mm in diameter. The fertilised female tunnels through the upper layers of the epidermis feeding on the liquid from the tissues it damages. It is within these tunnels that eggs are laid which produce six legged larvae that crawl to the surface of the skin. These larvae burrow into the skin forming pockets in which they mature then leave to seek a mate. The complete lifecycle takes between 17-21 days from egg to adult. In a mild infection scaly skin is observed with little hair loss, however in a chronic infection there is a thickening of the skin, hair loss, the formation of crusts and intense pruritus.

Infection appears to be acquired by direct contact with the skin so presumably the larval stage is the most likely to be infective.

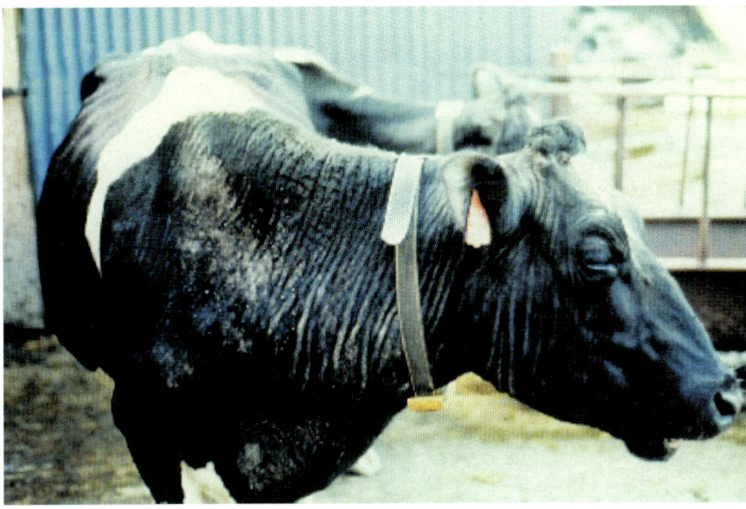

Sarcoptic mange-thickening of the skin and hair loss

Demodex bovis is a second burrowing mite although with less pathogenic properties than *Sarcoptes scabei* above, it has an elongated tapered body approximately 0.2mm in length as an adult. This mite has a predilection for sebaceous glands and hair follicles in which it completes its lifespan causing raised pea sized nodules containing caseous material and several thousand mites. It does however tend to burrow deeper into the dermis than *Sarcoptes scabei* and infection is thought to be acquired during feeding of the calf, limiting infection to the muzzle, head and back.

NON-BURROWING

Although a non-burrowing mite ***Psoroptes ovis*** does have severe pathogenic potential, this is due mainly to its pointed mouthparts and its feeding habits of piercing and chewing the surface of the skin. The adult is 0.75mm in length and the female can lay up to 90 eggs during her lifespan of 4-6 weeks, the growth from egg to larvae to nymph to adult takes approximately 10 days under optimum conditions. The feeding action produces initial vesicles the exudates from which produces a yellow centred crusty area that is moist at the borders where the mites breed. A chronic infection can be so debilitating that there can be a 20% reduction in feeding.

Chorioptes bovis feeds on surface debris and tends to only produce a mild flaky dermatitis near the tail in affected animals and has little pathogenic potential.

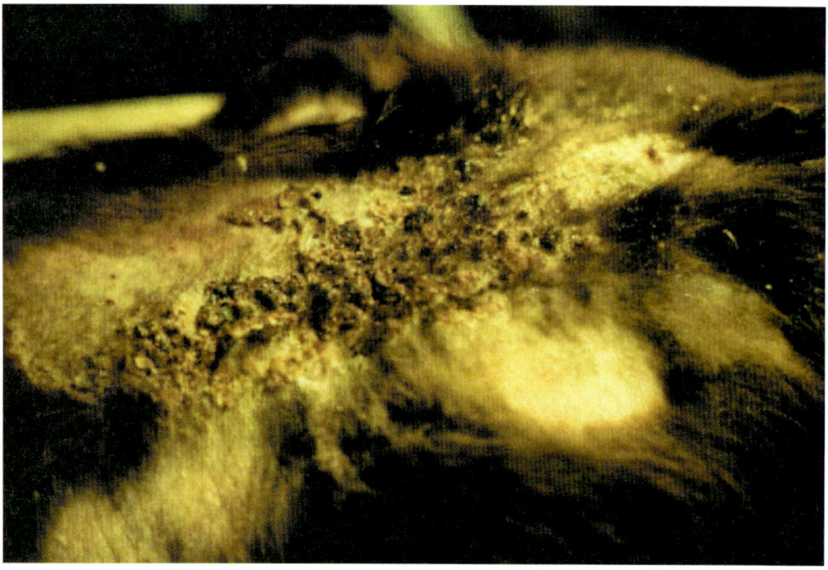

Psoroptes ovis mild infection

ZOONOTIC POTENTIAL

Sarcoptes scabei produces scabies in humans with itching, circular elevated skin lesions in areas that have contact with the animal such as the hands and wrists. Although the mites tend not to burrow in cases where infection is derived from an animal, the condition can lead to hypersensitivity in humans once affected.

4

NEOPLASIA

TUMOURS

INTRODUCTION

The term tumour literally applies to any abnormal swelling, but nowadays it tends to refer exclusively to neoplasms, which are abnormal new growth of tissue, in which cell multiplication is uncontrolled and progressive in addition to serving no purpose and growing faster than normal tissue. These neoplastic formations are classified as being either benign or malignant, the gross appearance of neoplasia is variable being dependant on their origin and type. Both malignant and benign tumours are served by increased blood vascularisation, any tumour requiring nutrients to continue growth. In the case of the rapidly growing malignant tumours the blood vessels tend to be thin and poorly formed and prone to rupture creating the appearance of haemorrhagic areas within the tumour.

BENIGN TUMOURS

These grow slowly, pushing aside normal tissue without invading it. They are usually encapsulated and do not normally produce secondary tumours within the body. Although some benign tumours are caused by viruses, on the whole they do not appear to be infectious. The effects of their presence tends to be physical, blockage of systems in the body and pressure applied to organs being obvious examples.

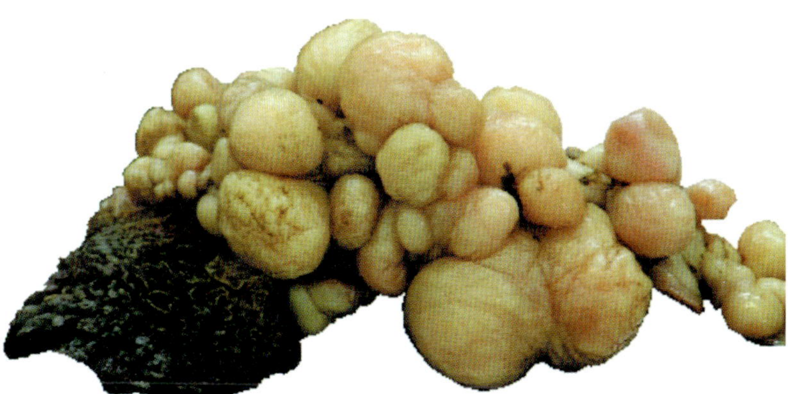

Fibro-papillomas in the oesophageal groove of the reticulum. Although benign, their presence can interfere with the process of rumination and lead to conditions such as bloat

MALIGNANT TUMOURS

Malignant tumours grow in an irregular shape and so quickly that the cell nutrition can become affected leading to cell death (necrosis) and ulceration. Malignant tumours invade surrounding tissue and can produce secondary tumours within the body through a process of metastasis (cells transported through the blood stream or lymphatic system.)

Tumours are further classified based upon the type of tissue cell from which the tumour cells originated. For example: Fibromas – composed of neoplastic fibrous cells, Lipomas – fat cells, Chondromas – cartilaginous cells, Osteomas – bone cells, Myelomas – blood cells, Adenomas – glandular cells etc. Tumours with the suffix sarcoma or carcinoma are malignant i.e. lymphosarcomas.

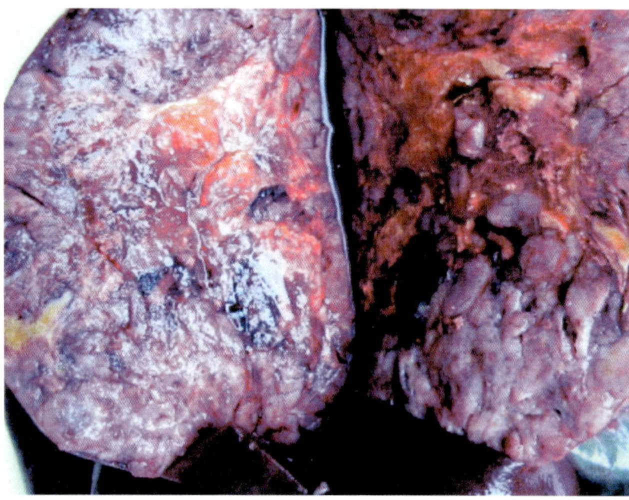

An incised lymphosarcomas, showing lobulation and haemorrhagic areas

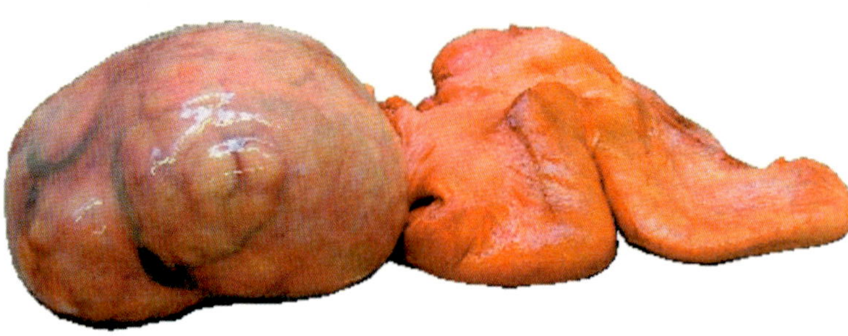

A large ovarian tumour

METASTASIS

This is the method of dissemination of malignant neoplasia throughout the body forming secondary tumours, the transfer of tumour cells tending to be either through direct contact between adjacent surfaces (contact spread) or via the blood or lymphatic circulation. Metastasis occurs as a product of the invasive abilities of malignant neoplasia, the detachment of tumour cells from the unencapsulated mass followed by infiltration of cells into surrounding tissue (contact), or erosion of the epithelial cells lining the blood and lymph vessels allowing ingress into the circulation. Studies have shown however that less than 1 in 10,000 neoplastic cells that enter these circulations will produce metastatic growth. As a general rule of thumb sarcomas are spread via the blood circulation and carcinomas via the lymphatics.

ENZOOTIC BOVINE LEUKOSIS

Enzootic bovine leukosis is a part of the bovine leukosis disease complex characterised by the formation of multiple malignant lymphosarcomas which also includes sporadic bovine leukosis. The latter condition is not attributable to an infectious agent and is generally associated with animals between 4 months and 2 years old. Enzootic bovine leukosis is caused by a retrovirus and occurs in animals over 1½ years of age, any multiple neoplasia in adult bovines should be reported in the UK where Enzootic Bovine Leukosis is a Notifiable Disease.

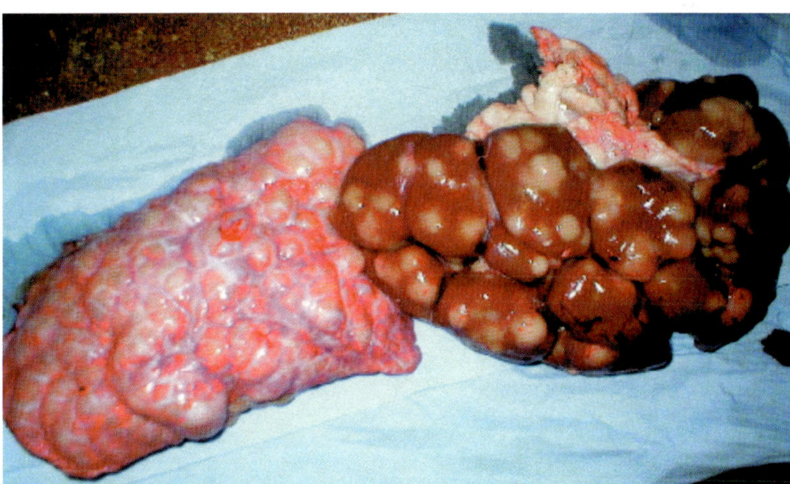

Enzootic bovine leukosis, multiple neoplasia in kidney and lung tissue

The EBL virus resists the action of the immune system by being an intracellular parasite of the lymphocytes, this also leads to infection being spread by blood contact including biting insects and inanimate objects such as injection needles and tattooing equipment.

Characteristics of Neoplasia

Benign tumours	Malignant tumours
Grow slowly	Rapid growth
Usually encapsulated	Unencapsulated
Do not invade local tissue	Highly invasive
No metastatic spread	Metastatic spread
Cut surface bland and homogenous	Variegated, haemorrhage and necrosis

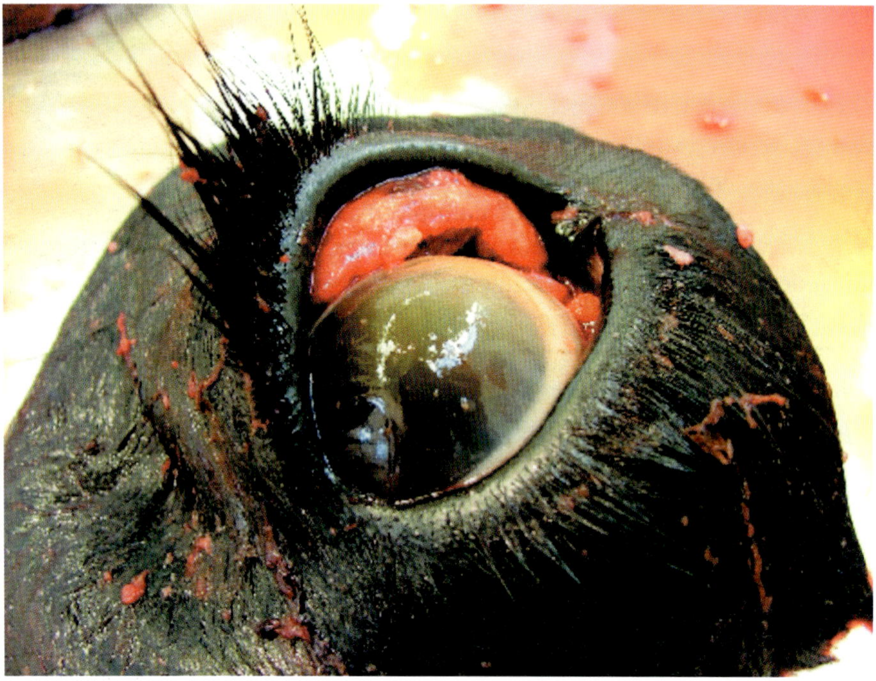

Neoplastic formation of the upper eyelid

5

CONDITIONS ENCOUNTERED AT BOVINE POST MORTEM INSPECTION

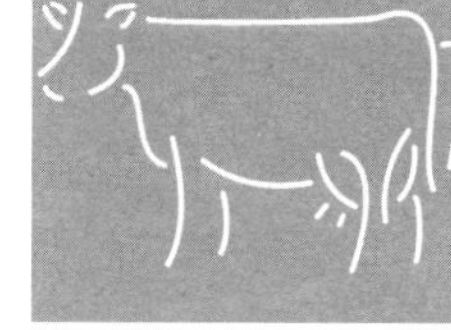

ABNORMAL ODOURS

Any abnormal odour in meat intensifies on heating, a fact utilised as a confirmatory test for uraemia, but this also renders the meat unmarketable and hence carcases and offal affected by abnormal odour / taste are rejected. The cause of an abnormal odour in cattle can be due to feed, medication or metabolic disorder.

Feed – "You are what you eat" is especially true in cattle, those slaughtered during the first week of being transferred to a turnip diet produce meat with a very distinct turnip odour. Cattle that have access to wild onions, leeks and garlic, as well as running the risk of toxin poisoning, will produce meat with a strong odour of these. Other foodstuffs that can cause abnormal odours include factory waste containing strong aromatic compounds such as orange rind.

Medication – Drugs or tonics administered before slaughter that include aromatic compounds such as aniseed, turpentine, linseed oil etc can taint the meat of that animal. The presence of medicinal smells, as well as rendering the carcase unfit for human consumption, may also prompt the taking of samples for laboratory analysis to ensure that relevant drug withdrawal periods have been met.

Metabolic disorder – cattle can be affected by acetonaemia or ketosis when fevered or after giving birth or late in their pregnancy. It is generally accepted that this is due to ketones produced when body fat is broken down to produce energy. These ketones are reabsorbed into the blood circulation and then into the body tissue. The carcase smells strongly of 'nail varnish', a smell that becomes more pronounced when the tissue is heated.

Carcases with an abnormal odour or taste are rejected as unfit for human consumption

ABSCESSES

An abscess is a collection of pus surrounded by fibrous tissue; it is part of the bodies' defence mechanism normally triggered by the presence of pus forming bacteria. This fibrous tissue is a normal healthy reaction and consists of newly formed connective tissue and blood vessels. Pus may consist of dead or dying bacteria, dead tissue cells that formerly occupied the area, dead or dying white blood cells, debris and a certain amount of fluid exuded from the blood vessels in the vicinity.

If the organisms multiply, the abscess will continue to increase in size until the pus escapes. If the abscess is near the surface of tissue part of the wall becomes necrotic and is removed allowing the pus to discharge. If the abscess is deeper within tissue and the pus is under tension it can burrow through less resistant tissue and reach the surface through a canal known as a sinus.

If the bodies' immune response is sufficient to destroy the organisms contained in the pus the abscess may remain localised and be eventually absorbed, caseated or calcified.

Intramuscular abscesses are generally caused by injection, the use of unsterilised needles introducing infection through the skin. If localised the affected area is trimmed and rejected as unfit for human consumption. Cattle, especially barley fed beef are prone to abscesses in the liver (hepatic). If present the liver is rejected.

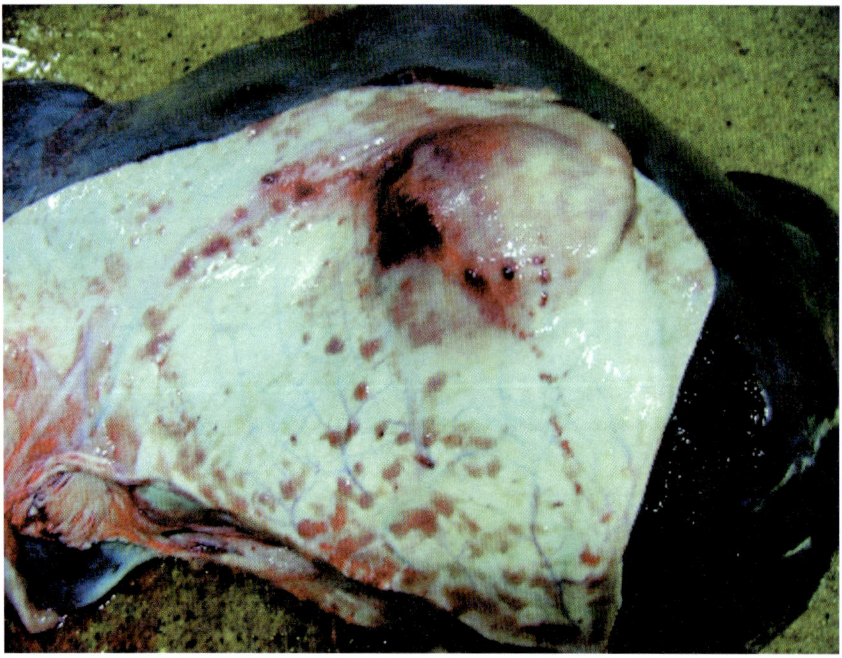

A large hepatic abscess adhering to the diaphragm and setting up parietal pleurisy

If the infection is not contained, it can lead to pyaemia, which warrants the rejection of the whole carcase and associated offal.

The trimming of localised abscesses affects the carcase quality, especially when removed from commercially higher value cuts of meat such as the legs.

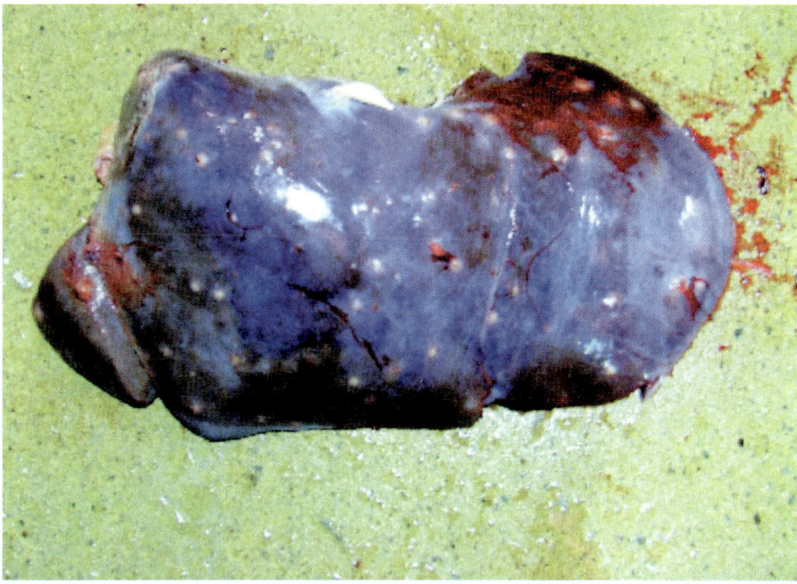

Multiple abscesses in a bovine liver

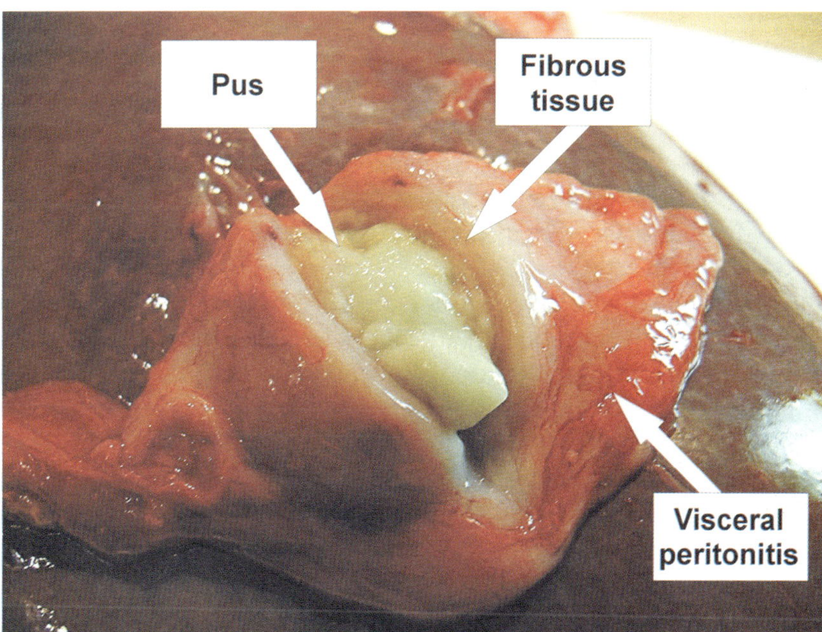

Anatomy of a hepatic abscess

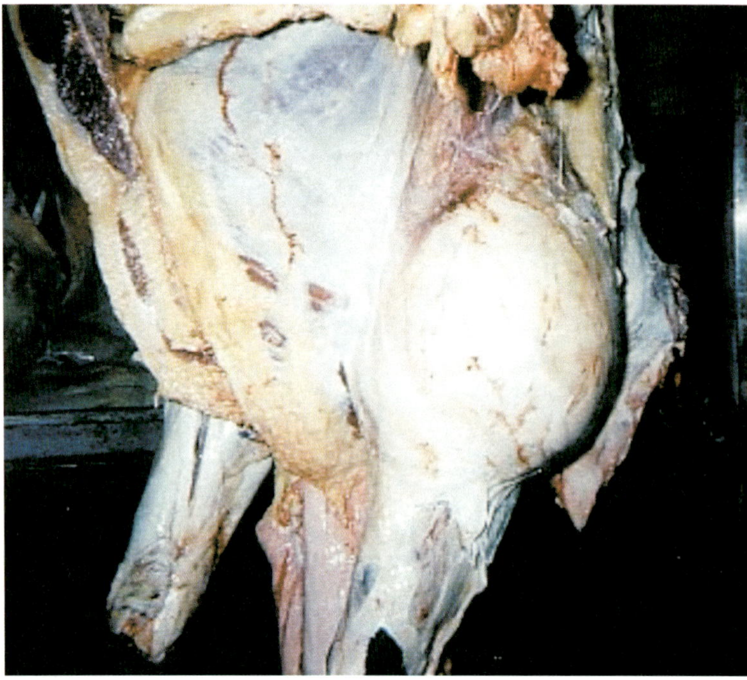

A large abscess on the foreleg of an over thirty month bullock

PYAEMIA / GENERALISED ABSCESSATION

This condition is produced when pyogenic (pus forming) bacteria gain access to the blood stream and form abscesses throughout the body. Access to the bloodstream is normally from a suppurative focus such as injection abscesses, injury, etc.

In the live animal high fever and the presence of an area of local infection may be apparent. If the infection is particularly virulent it can cause the animals' death. In young animals the route of infection can be through the infection of the umbilicus.

Acute pyaemia exhibits lesions in the carcase similar to those of septicaemia, with the addition of abscesses. The presence of abscesses throughout the carcase especially in conjunction with a localised infection warrants complete rejection of the carcase and offal.

Navel ill, or umbilical pyaemia, occurs as a result of bacterial infection of the umbilicus, which becomes thickened and full of pus. The infection can spread from the umbilicus to the liver, producing abscesses, which would warrant rejection of the liver.

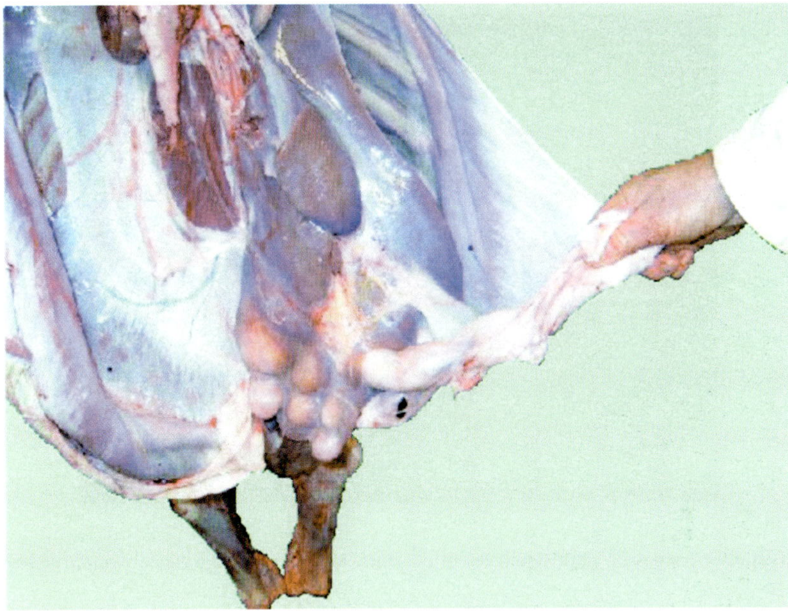

Umbilical pyaemia in a calf. Note multiple hepatic abscesses and pus filled umbilicus

If there are signs that the infection has travelled further, become systemic, (abscesses in other organs, small pin-point haemorrhages – petechiae - in the kidneys, joint ill) the carcase and associated offal are rejected as unfit for human consumption.

ACTINOBACILLOSIS

Actinobacillosis, also known as 'wooden tongue' is caused by a bacterium *Actinobacillus ligniersi*. The term 'wooden tongue' describes the chronic form where there is an increase in fibrous tissue in the tongue reducing flexibility. Typically *A. ligniersi* produces small abscesses joined by extensive connective tissue, affecting areas up to 1cm in diameter.

The infection is spread by the lymphatic system and can affect other soft tissues, especially the lymph nodes of the head. The pus is a bright yellow, sometimes orange and is granular, which can be felt when incising the area.

In chronic infections, other areas of the carcase may be affected, including the liver and the reticulum, which are affected by a glistening, white, fibrous tissue.

It is important to differentiate the nodules produced by actinobacillosis from those of tuberculosis, the basic differences being:

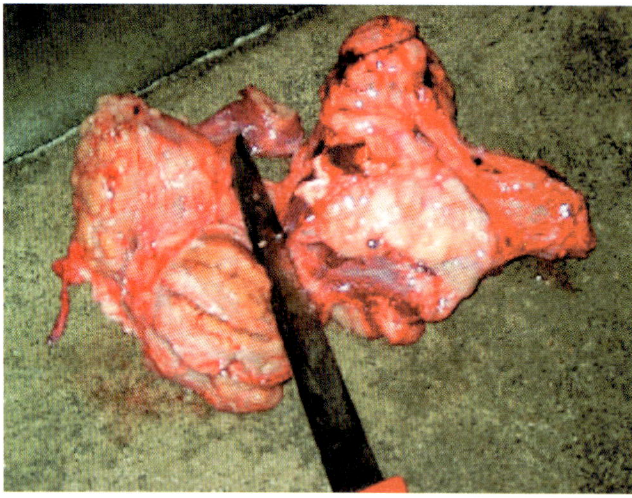

Granular lesions of actinobacillosis in enlarged bovine retropharyngeal lymph nodes

- Actinobacillosis nodules contain granular pus, those of tuberculosis do not.
- Actinobacillosis nodules tend to protrude, those of tuberculosis do not.
- Actinobacillosis lesions do not calcify, tuberculous lesions do.

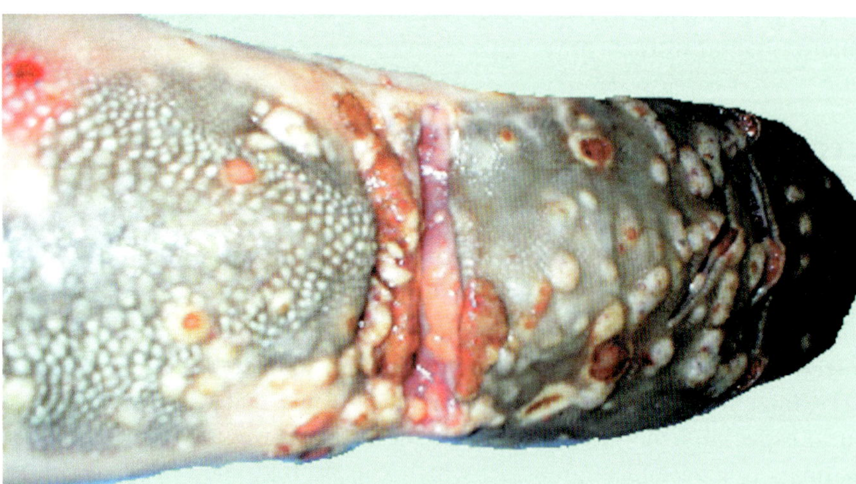

Actinobacillosis in a bovine tongue

If there is any doubt in these cases, the lesions must be treated as tuberculous.

Organs affected with actinobacillosis are rejected as unfit for human consumption. If the condition is generalised throughout the carcase, both the entire carcase and associated offal are rejected as unfit for human consumption.

ACTINOMYCOSIS

Actinomycosis, also known as 'lumpy jaw' is caused by a bacterium *Actinomyces bovis*. It is a disease that affects the bones of the head, especially those of the mandible.

The mandible becomes thickened and enlarged due to the formation of multiple small abscesses giving a honeycombed appearance when the bone is cut. Actinomycosis does not normally spread to the lymph nodes of the head.

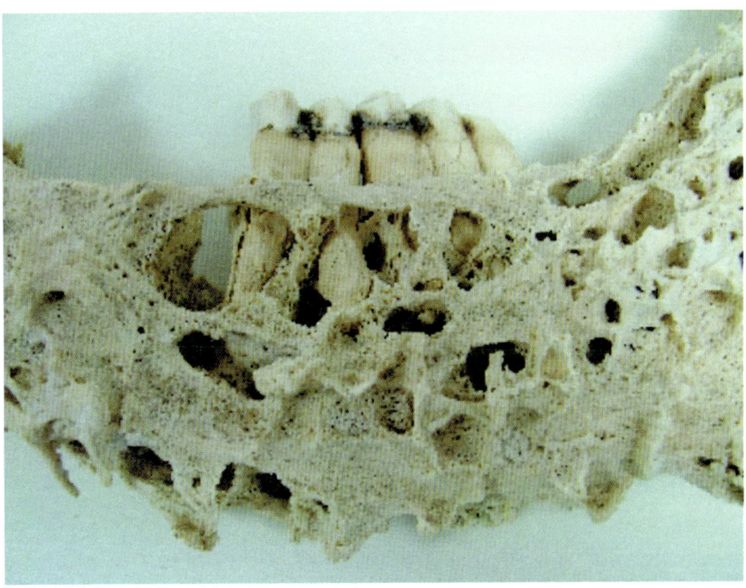

A typical 'honeycomb' mandible

In the live animal actinomycosis can cause the teeth to loosen and eating becomes difficult. In the chronic form the infection can spread to the bones of the sinus causing difficulty in breathing. Actinomycosis abscesses do 'track' (fistulate) to the surface so pus can be observed on the skin, the tracks leaving small scars when they recede.

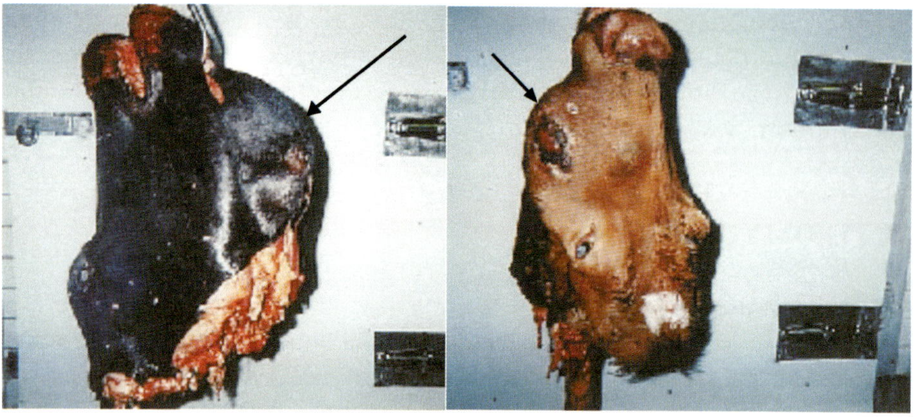

Actinomycosis of mandible and upper jaw respectively

Affected parts are rejected.

ANAEMIA

This is defined as a deficiency in the blood such as the number and size of the red blood cells or the quantity of haemoglobin in the blood. This may be due to haemorrhage, the presence of internal or external parasites, chronic illness, iron deficiency, bracken poisoning or in the case of aplastic anaemia, where the body ceases production of red blood cells, it may be drug induced.

Anaemia is difficult to detect in the live animal, which may show signs of breathlessness, loss of energy and appetite and have pale mucous membranes.

An anaemic carcase is generally pale in colour, and is often emaciated, warranting rejection of the entire carcase and associated offals.

ARTHRITIS

Arthritis is inflammation of the structures of joints between bones. Arthritis may be infectious, traumatic or non-infectious.

The synovial joints, knee, knuckles, shoulder, provide a nutrient rich fluid surrounded by a good blood supply that offers ideal conditions for bacterial growth. Microorganisms may enter the joint through a penetrative wound, via the blood stream or from a nearby area of infection, foot rot for example.

When infected the joint swells as fluid increases, the synovial membrane becomes thicker (fibrinous). If the infection enters the blood stream it can lead to polyarthritis, where most joints are infected, especially the large joints of the limbs.

At post mortem inspection enlarged joints are opened and examined.

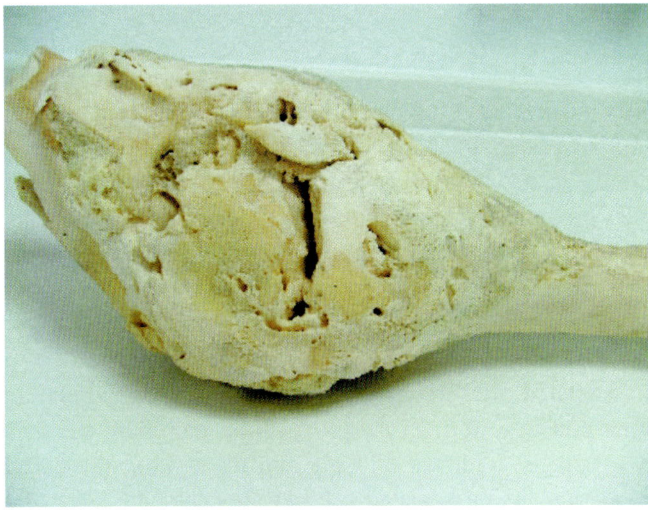

Osteoarthritis in a joint

All cases of septic polyarthritis warrants rejection of the entire carcase and offal, as the infection is spread by the bloodstream and is said to be systemic, the synovial fluid resembles a 'beaten egg' and contains pus, blood and other turbid matter, and is associated with septicaemia, pyaemia or emaciation.

In other forms of arthritis the rest of the carcase, organs and lymph nodes are inspected for evidence of a generalised infection which if present warrants rejection of the carcase and offal. The affected area of inflammation is trimmed if localised.

BLACKLEG / GANGRENE

Gangrene denotes a two-stage condition, bacterial invasion and putrefaction following death of body tissue (necrosis), normally through loss of nutrition to an area. It is associated with fever, pain and an extremely unpleasant odour. There are various forms of gangrene which include:

Dry gangrene – a gradual condition, usually found at the extremities of the body and involves no secondary bacterial infection. This is due to a slow decrease in blood supply to the area. The tissues become dry and black and shrivel. The affected area has a definite border at the point where the blood supply continues.

Moist gangrene- a sudden cessation of blood to an area causing rapid death to tissues. This form shows as a swollen, usually blistered area that spreads rapidly due to toxins formed in the affected tissue causing necrosis in neighbouring tissue.

Gas gangrene – also known as emphysematous gangrene, an acute condition such as blackleg involving species of Clostridrial bacteria. This takes the form of a swelling usually in the large muscles of the leg and forequarter that crackles like paper when pressed. On inspection the affected area is dry and sponge-like with a rancid smell. The centre of the area is dry and the muscles are bluish-black, the edges of the affected area are usually wet, other tissue is yellow and jelly-like.

Carcases and associated offal in cases of blackleg or gas gangrene are rejected as unfit for human consumption. In cases of moist gangrene the affected part is rejected unless there is evidence of toxaemia throughout the carcase in which case the entire carcase and associated offal are rejected. In cases of localised dry gangrene the affected area is rejected.

CIRRHOSIS

Cirrhosis is the term used to describe the change of state of the liver substance due to the presence and formation of fibrous connective tissue, which can result in distortion of the liver shape. Cirrhosis of the liver can also lead to jaundice.

The production of this fibrous tissue is part of the bodies defence system, the tissue having been produced as a repair to injury (trauma) to the liver cells. This trauma can be caused by parasitic infestation, for example the migration of immature liver flukes through the liver, which tends to be most common cause of cirrhosis in cattle, however, it can also be due to toxins, certain strains of moulds such as penicillin and through the ingestion of certain plants.

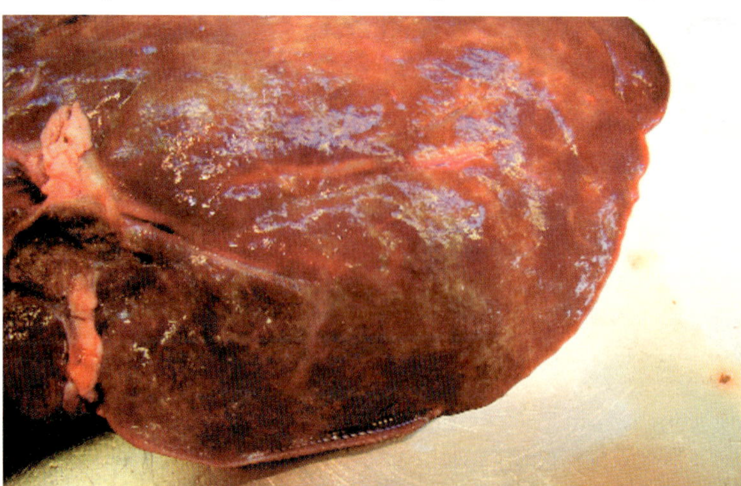

Cirrhosis of the liver due to *Fasciola hepatic*a larvae migration

Cirrhotic livers are rejected as unfit for human consumption.

EMPHYSEMA

Emphysema is an accumulation of air, or gas in tissues. This can take the form of subcutaneous emphysema as occurs in conditions such as gas gangrene. This rejection condition, however, refers to pulmonary emphysema, where the lungs are distended due to air escaping from the alveoli (the terminal ends of the bronchioles), known as alveolar emphysema, or the escape of air into the lung tissue itself, interstitial emphysema.

Interstitial emphysema can be observed on inspection as a marked accentuation of the lobular texture of the lungs, and can even extend through the lung tissue to the area between the lungs and their membrane covering, the pleura.

Lungs affected with emphysema are rejected as unfit for human consumption. This is due to the fact that the primary cause of emphysema is an obstruction of the airflow in the affected area, which can be due to objects inhaled, but more commonly it is secondary to another condition such as bronchitis or tuberculosis. The air may also contain pathogenic bacteria.

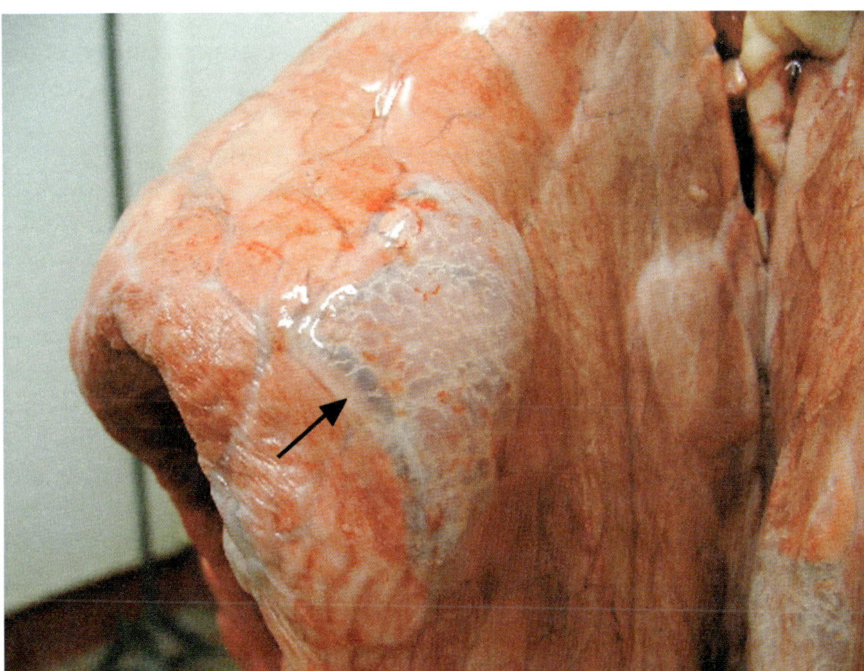

Detail of emphysema in the cardiac lobe

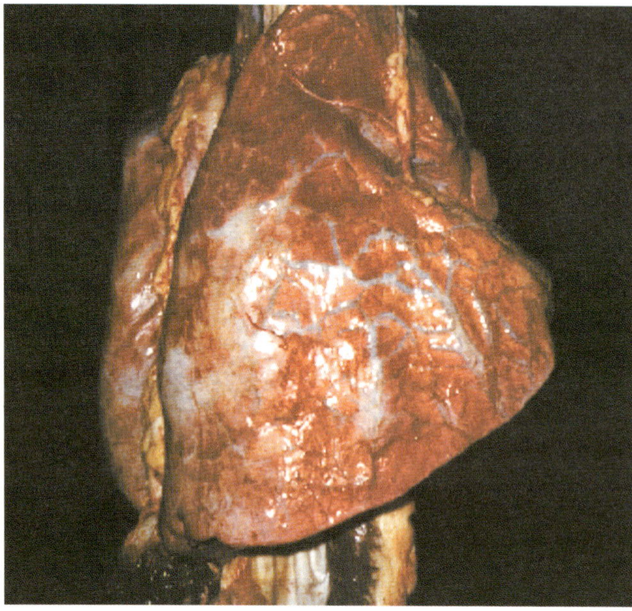

Interstitial emphysema

ENTERITIS

Enteritis is inflammation of the intestines. It can be either acute or chronic and occurs during the course of some diseases, as a result of the action of parasites or toxic agent.

In the live animal enteritis is characterised by diarrhoea.

At post mortem inspection with acute enteritis the stomach and intestinal contents are often blood stained. The mesenteric lymph nodes are enlarged and haemorrhagic. The liver shows signs of pathological change (fatty degeneration) and the gall bladder is often thickened. The lungs can be hepatised, the lung substance altering to give the appearance of liver, and small haemorrhages (petechiae) are found in the kidneys.

With chronic enteritis there are areas of tissue death (necrosis), especially in the intestines at the caecum and colon. The bowel wall can be thickened with greenish yellow necrotic material. In cases of chronic enteritis the carcase is examined for signs of systemic infection.

Jöhne's disease is a chronic infection of the lower intestine causing thickening and eventual corrugation, (see separate entry in Section Two – Diseases of Cattle)

If the carcase shows signs of acute enteritis, both the entire carcase and associated offal are rejected as unfit for human consumption.

If the carcase displays lesions that indicate chronic enteritis the affected parts are rejected, unless evidence of systemic infection warrants rejection of the entire carcase and offal as unfit for human consumption.

FEVER

This encompasses fever, toxaemia and septicaemia. The carcase is fiery in appearance, has usually bled badly, the carcase lymph nodes are enlarged and have undergone change.

TOXAEMIA

This is the presence of bacterial toxins in the bloodstream of the animal. If these toxins have produced generalised and systemic changes within the carcase the carcase is considered unfit for human consumption and is rejected. These changes may take the form of cloudy swelling or fatty change in the liver, kidneys or heart muscles.

SEPTICAEMIA

This is the presence of, and multiplication of, bacteria in the bloodstream of the animal. This differs from the condition of bacteraemia in that the organisms are widely distributed as is the subsequent tissue damage, and the organisms are not only present in the blood but are actively multiplying therein.

The affected carcase is congested, bleeds badly and rigor mortis is slight or absent. Small haemorrhages known as petechial haemorrhages are present in organs such as the kidneys. The lymph nodes are enlarged; the livers and kidneys can undergo pathological change.

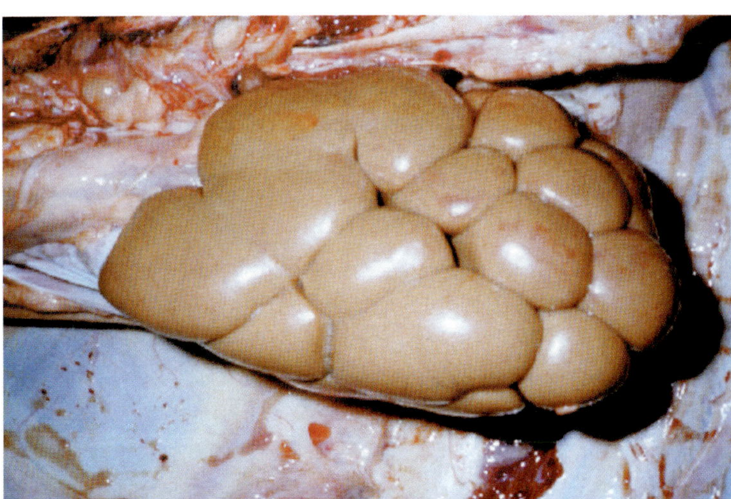

A kidney from a septicaemic carcase.

Fevered, septicaemic and toxaemic carcases are rejected as unfit for human consumption. The congestion of the carcase affects the keeping quality of the meat, rendering it unmarketable, but more importantly the causal organisms may be pathogenic, which would render the consumption of the carcase dangerous to the consumer. Therefore in cases where the carcase displays signs of the above conditions the benefit of doubt must always be given to the consumer.

Studies have shown that flesh from animals suffering from generalised septic conditions; especially those of the intestinal tract are most likely to give rise to gastro-intestinal disturbances in man.

JAUNDICE

Jaundice, or icterus, is a condition where the tissue of the body are coloured yellow, this colouration being a symptom of bile pigments (bilirubin – yellow/orange and biliverdin – green) being present in the circulating blood.

The presence of bile pigments in the blood results from conditions affecting the functioning of the liver or the blood. The affects on the liver can be due to toxins (toxic jaundice), blockage of the bile ducts of the liver by calculi (stones) or parasites such as liver fluke (obstructive jaundice). A reduction in the number of red blood cells (haemolytic icterus) can occur in certain diseases such as Redwater fever.

The yellow colouration can be most easily discerned in the white tissues of the body (eyes, internal mouth, tendons, fat and cartilage for example.) Yellow discolouration of fat may occur due to problems in breaking down carotene and xanthophylls found in grass, however in practice this will not discolour cartilage and incision through the xiphoid cartilage at the end of the sternum (brisket) will appear white in these cases.

In cases of doubt the carcase is examined in natural daylight, as the jaundice is more easily discernible than under artificial light. There is also a chemical test, the Rimmington and Fowrie test that will differentiate between carotene and bile salts in fat.

Jaundiced carcases and their associated offal are rejected as unfit for human consumption. Carotene pigmentation (confined solely to the fat) as is seen in Jersey and Guernsey cattle is passed as fit for human consumption

MASTITIS

Mastitis is inflammation of the udder. If encountered the udder is rejected. The main importance of mastitis is that the normal causative organisms *Pasteurella haemolytica* and *Staphylococcus aureus* are pus-forming bacteria. If these bacteria are not successfully contained within the udder access can be gained to the rest of the animal, resulting in secondary abscess formation, pyaemia and septicaemia, all of which warrant rejection of the entire carcase and offal as unfit for human consumption. Septic mastitis can lead to gangrene.

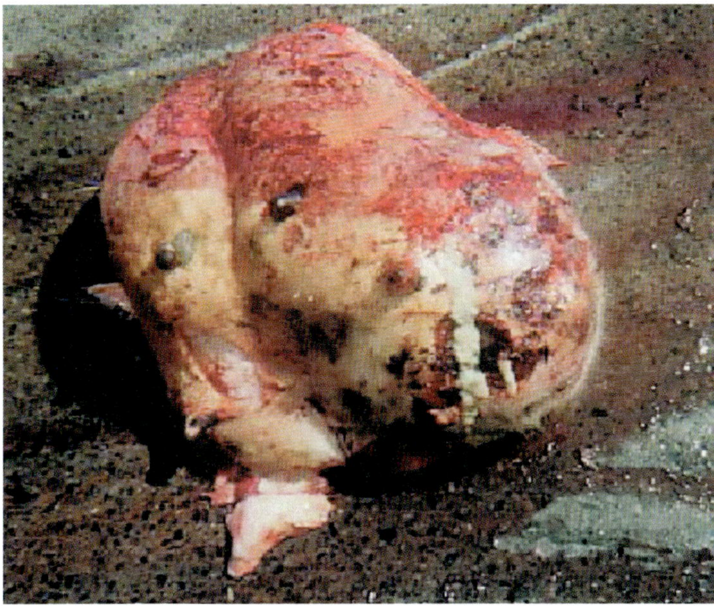

An enlarged, firm udder oozing pus, the carcase was passed as there were no signs of systemic spread or emaciation

MELANOSIS

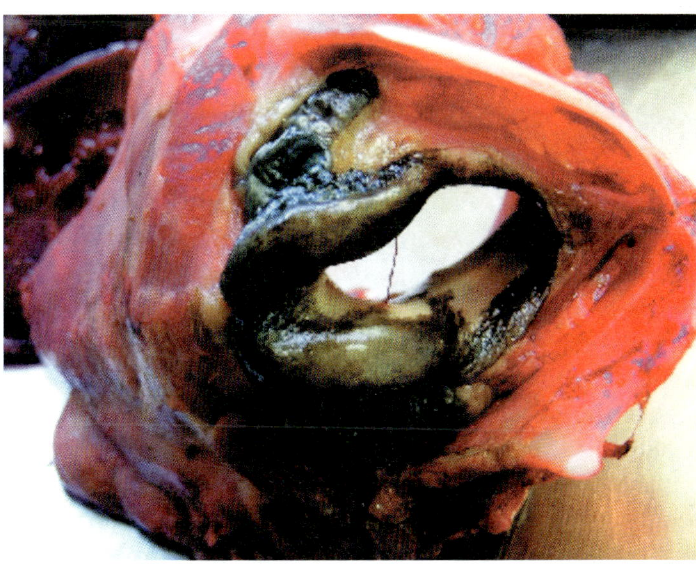

Melanosis in a larynx. Common in Jersey cattle

Melanin is a normal protein based pigment of the body, which colours the horns, hair, palate etc of cattle. It can occur in abnormal amounts within the body, especially tissues such as the lungs, kidneys and spinal cord in the latter case it is also known as 'black pith'. These deposits are jet black, varying in size and shape and normally resemble ink splashes. Melanosis is congenital and the deposits are laid down in the foetus. Affected parts are rejected.

If the pigmentation is generalised throughout the muscular tissue the entire carcase is condemned.

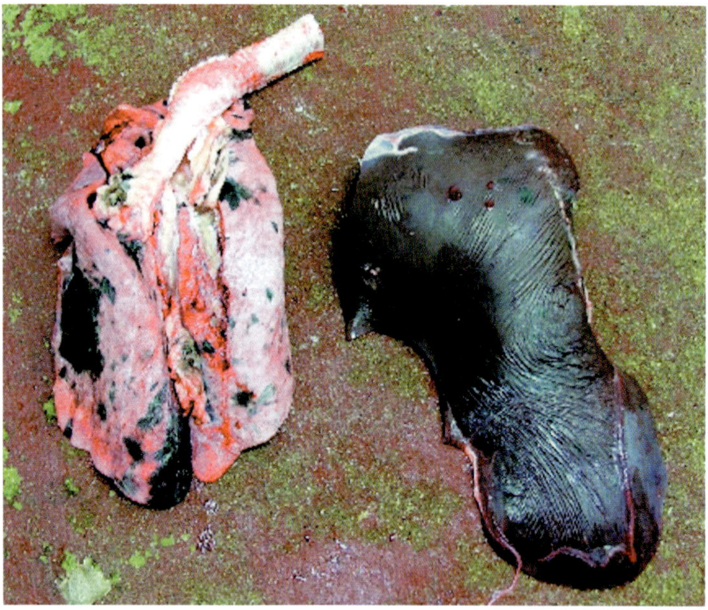

Melanosis in lung tissue and liver

METRITIS

Metritis is inflammation of the uterus, and generally occurs as one of three types.

Septic metritis is a bacterial infection and normally results from problems during birthing, such as retention of the placenta, rupture or injury to the uterine mucous membrane, and very rarely due to the reabsorbtion of the foetus before birth.

The live animal suffers high fever, increased pulse rate, muscular weakness and frequently the inability to rise.

At inspection the uterus is enlarged up to three times normal size and is full of foul smelling chocolate or greyish fluid. The internal membrane of the uterus is thickened and discoloured, and the external surface may exhibit peritonitis. Toxaemia can be produced within the carcase, with enlargement of the lymph nodes.

Carcases showing lesions indicating acute septic metritis are rejected as unfit for human consumption.

Chronic endometritis is characterised by a purulent vaginal discharge but no signs of fever or physiological disturbance. The uterus is rejected.

Pyometra (pus in the uterus) occurs without systemic infection of the carcase. The uterus is rejected, although in chronic form this can lead to emaciation of the carcase that could warrant the rejection of the entire carcase and associated offal.

MUSCLE DEGENERATION

The muscle cells of any animal can alter type due to various reasons, ranging from an increase in fat to the altering of the tissue type to bone. This degeneration or fibrosis can occur due to various stimuli, genetic susceptibility, injury (trauma), and nutritional deficiency.

Muscular fibrosis – (interstitial fibrosis) occurs where normal tissue is replaced by white, fibrous connective tissue. This is normally due to trauma that has damaged cells within the muscle.

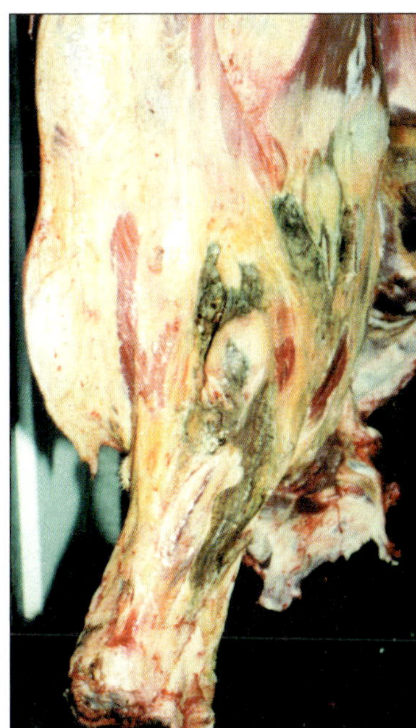

Muscle necrosis following trauma

Muscular steatosis – steatosis is the change of any cell to a fat cell (adipose cell). This can occur throughout the musculature but in cattle is most commonly seen in presternal calcification due to repetitive damage to the brisket, a condition also known as 'putty brisket.'

Atrophy – muscle degeneration through cell death (necrosis), normally occurring due to damage to the nerves supplying the muscle resulting in lack of stimuli and subsequent use. In all cases of muscle degeneration or fibrosis the affected part is rejected as unfit for human consumption. If the condition is generalised throughout the carcase (as can occur in White Muscle Disease) the entire carcase is rejected.

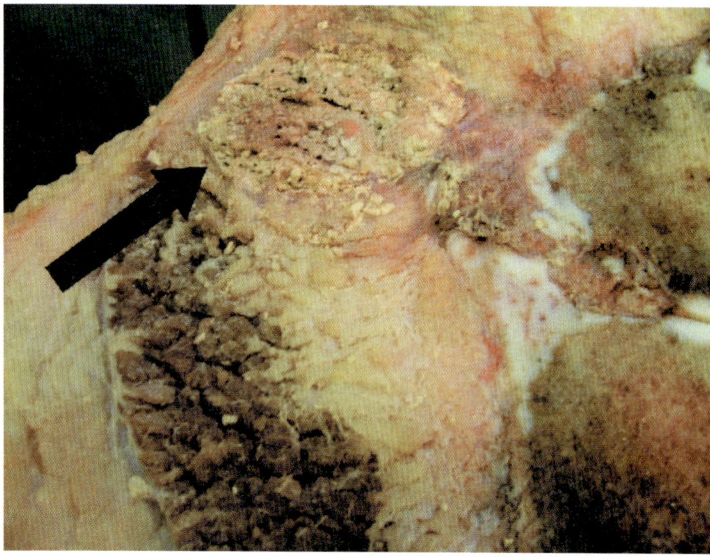

Presternal calcification (arrowed)

Myopathy – also known as White Muscle Disease. This can range from light coloured patches in the muscle to white streaks. There are various causes of this, but in cattle it is predominantly a nutritional myopathy, due to selenium or vitamin E deficiency. The heart muscle is frequently affected. Other causes are genetic (genetic myopathy) and due to toxins (toxic myopathy.)

NEPHRITIS / NEPHROSIS

Nephritis denotes inflammation of the kidney. Nephrosis denotes the change of state of the kidney.

The basic function of the kidneys is the excretion of waste materials from the blood stream and the maintenance of the blood water proportions. Urine is passed through two ureters to the bladder. As the structure of the kidney is basically made up of filtration systems (nephrons) the kidneys are susceptible to infection from various sources and are examined closely at inspection, some of the conditions encountered are:

Pyelonephritis, which occurs when pus-forming organisms gain entry either through the blood stream (pyaemia) or from a rising infection from the bladder (cystitis). If one side is affected (unilateral) the affected organ is rejected after examination of the rest of the carcass. If both kidneys are affected (bilateral infection) the carcase may be rejected depending on evidence of a systemic infection.

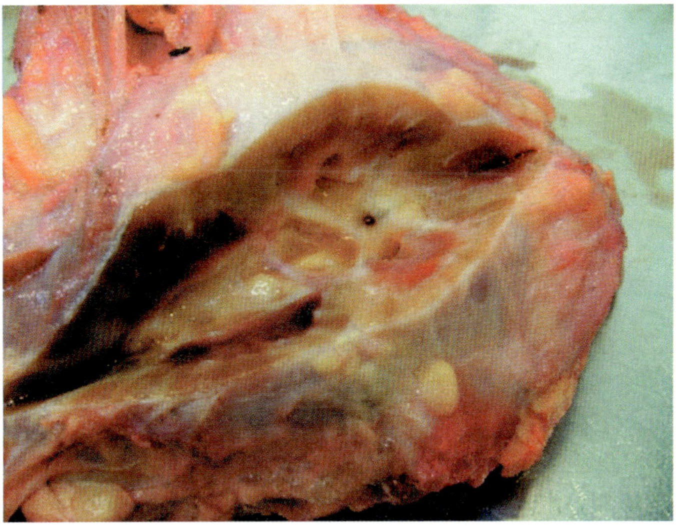

Nephrosis

Hydronephrosis occurs as a blockage of one or both ureters preventing urine from draining to the bladder. If unilateral the kidney is rejected. If bilateral the carcase is examined for uraemia (reabsorbtion of urine into the blood) and may be rejected as unfit for human consumption.

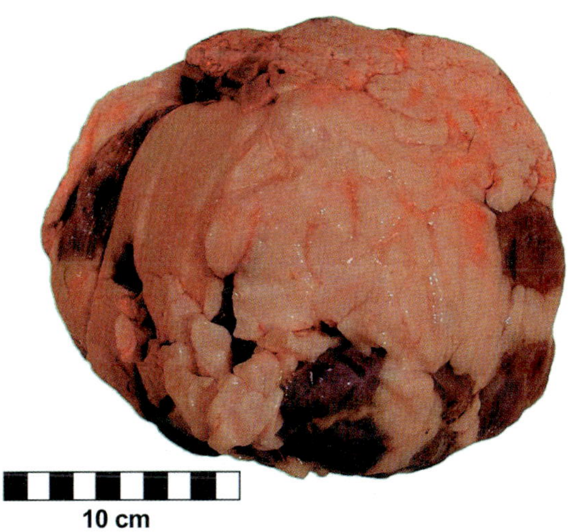

An enlarged kidney with hydronephrosis

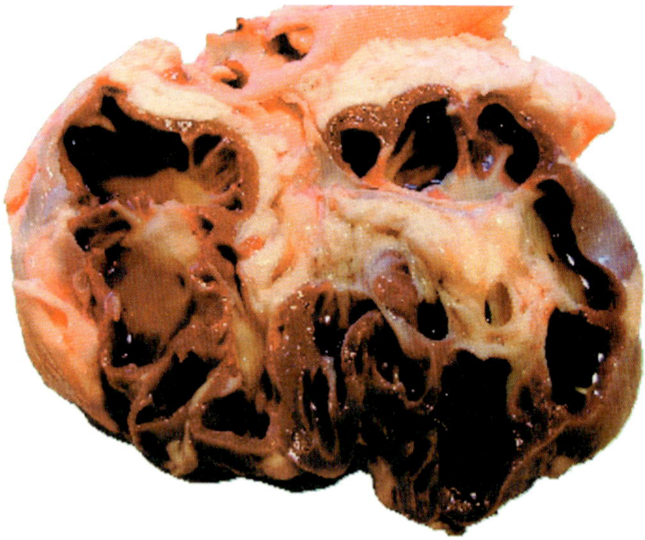

A section through the kidney illustrating destruction of kidney tissue

Fibroplastic nephritis or white spotted kidney occurs exclusively in young calves. This takes the form of small, pale, circular nodules within the cortex of the kidneys. These nodules vary in size up to approximately 6mm in diameter. It is thought that they are possibly due to an *E.coli* infection and disappear as the calf grows older. One or both kidneys may be involved, the affected kidney is rejected.

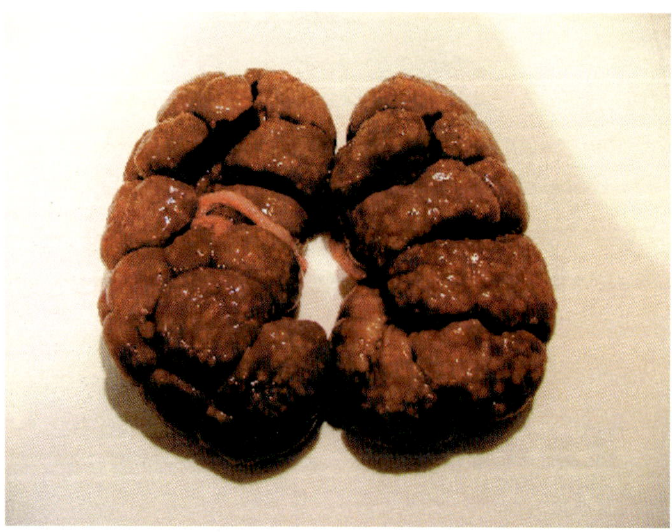

Fibroplastic nephritis

The kidneys are also prone to infarction, whereby the blood supply to the cortex is obstructed by an embolus and this results in the death (necrosis) of the cells supplied by that blood vessel. In the kidney these appear as pale spots on the surface and have a characteristic cone shape when the kidney is incised. These kidneys are rejected as unfit for human consumption.

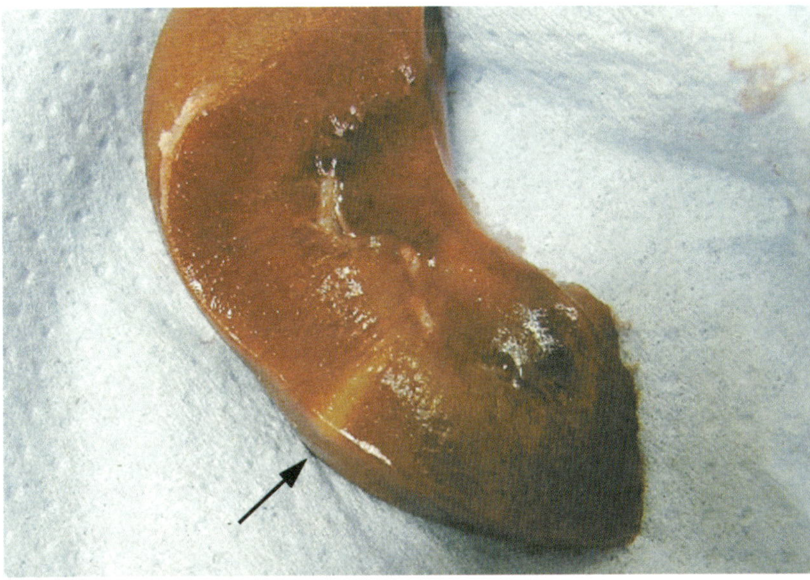

A section through a kidney lobule illustrating a typical wedge shaped infarct

Renal Uroliths. The formation of kidney stones (uroliths) is normally due to metabolic imbalance within the body forcing the deposition of salts of calcium, phosphorus or magnesium within the cortex of the kidneys. The concentration of these salts in the urine is finely balanced; precipitation of these salts from the urine to form insoluble material can be prompted by the presence of dead cells or pus foci in infected kidneys in addition to an imbalance of these minerals within the diet. Eventually the salt builds up into concentric layers around the initial deposition forming balls which can lead to blockage of the ureters before it leaves the kidney. During this time the kidney still operates as usual, removing nitrogenous waste from the blood, unable to escape this fluid builds up destroying the kidney tissue. When this condition is produced by a dietary imbalance there is always a distinct possibility that it can become a bilateral infection at which point uraemia should be considered.

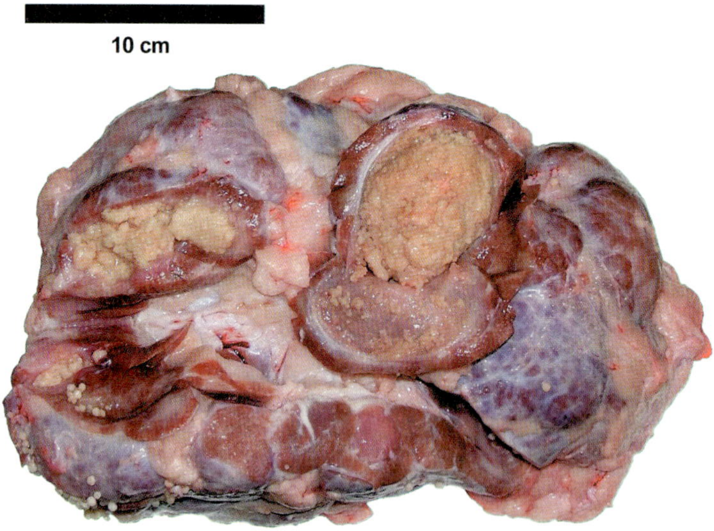

A grossly enlarged kidney containing uroliths

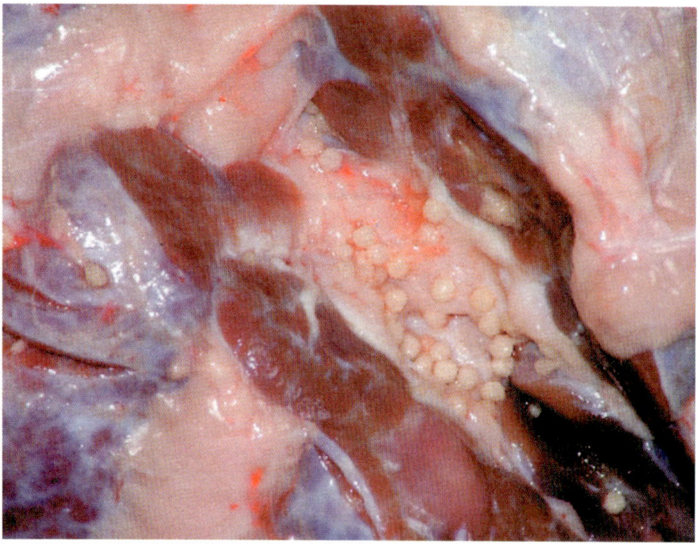

Detail of renal calculi

Genetic cysts, Retention cysts

These cysts tend to affect only a single lobule or partial lobule of the kidney. They are not felt to be due to a pathological cause but a congenital defect in the tubule supplying the affected area. As such the unaffected areas are considered fit for human consumption. These cysts are often accompanied by hypertrophic growth in the remaining kidney tissue.

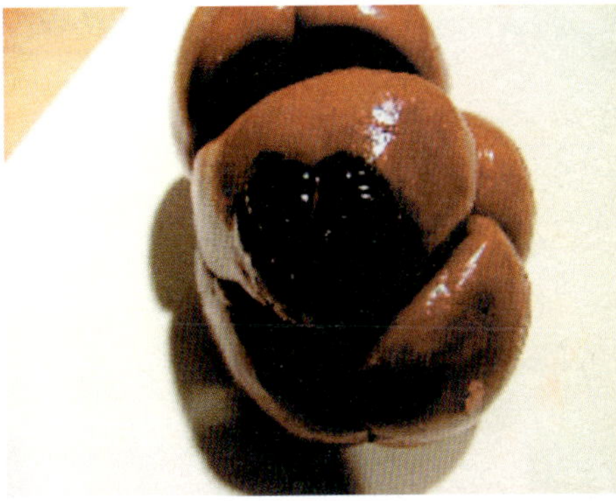

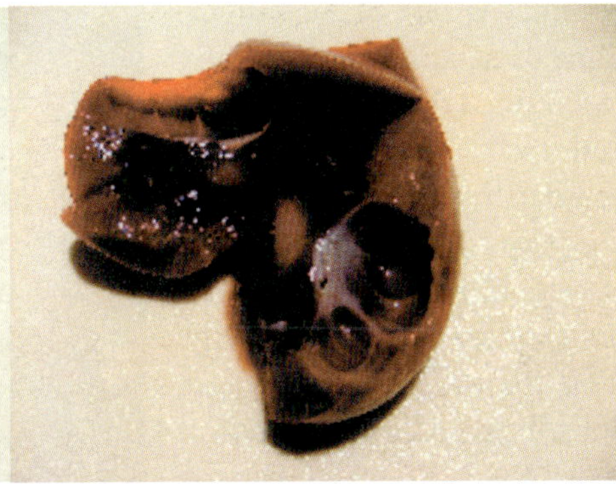

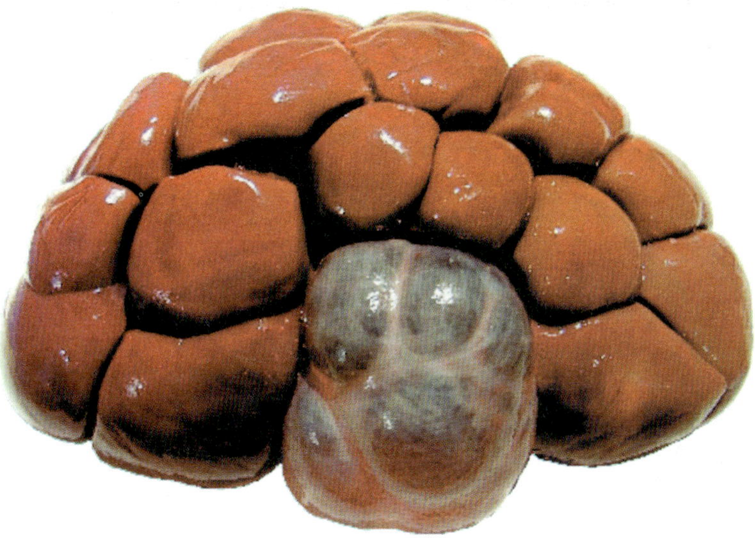

A retention cyst affecting a single lobule of the kidney

OEDEMA AND EMACIATION

Emaciation is generally due to a pathological condition. The muscle wastes and the remaining fat becomes jelly like. The flesh is wet and does not set. In contrast a similar condition, poorness, is due to a change in the functioning of the animal, such as shortage of food etc.

Emaciated carcases that are considered borderline cases are detained overnight. Those that are emaciated do not set, and generally become wetter.

Emaciated carcases are rejected as unfit for human consumption.

Oedema is a general term describing the accumulation of fluid within the body; this fluid accumulation is brought about by a dysfunction of the body system. Bottle jaw, fluid under the area of the lower jaw (submandibular oedema) is one of the clinical signs of acute Fascioliasis, for example. Hydropericardium denotes fluid in the pericardium, hydrothorax indicates fluid in the chest cavity and ascites describes fluid in the abdominal cavity.

If the oedema is localised, the affected area is rejected. If generalised the whole carcase and associated offal are rejected as unfit for human consumption. Emaciated carcases are very often associated with generalised oedema.

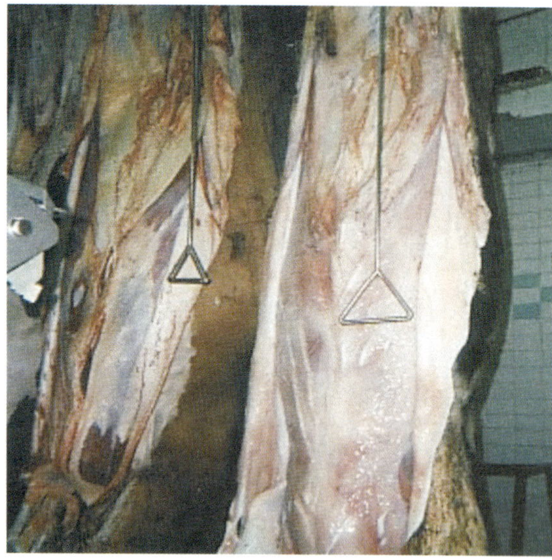

An oedematous carcase on the right. Note the obvious wetness and transparency of the subcutaneous fat.

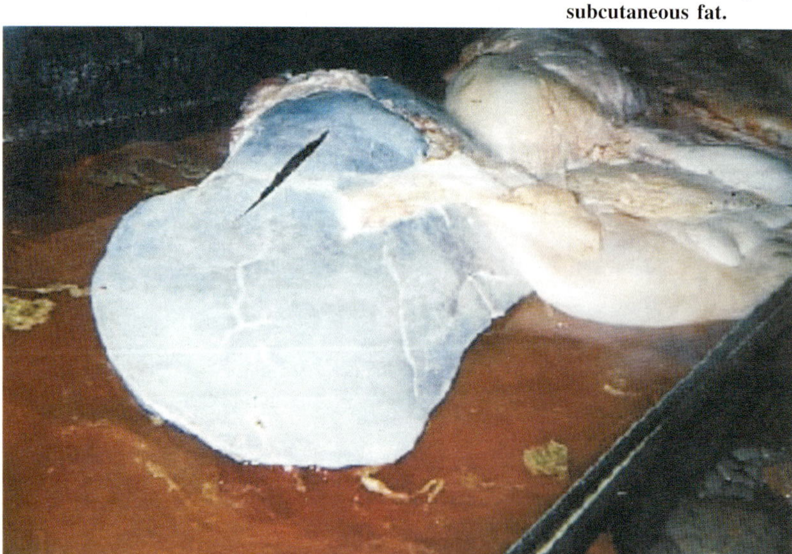

Offal from the carcase pictured. Notice the cooked appearance of the liver and state of the intestines

PERICARDITIS

Pericarditis is the inflammation of the pericardium, causing it to become thickened, opaque and in some cases adherent to the surface of the heart. The clear fluid contained within the pericardium can become straw coloured and contain clots of greyish white fibrin.

The cause of pericarditis can be traumatic, where the pericardium is penetrated by a foreign object, as can occur in cases of Traumatic Reticulitis, it can also be bacterial in origin, as in the case of tuberculosis or be due to simple non-specific causes.

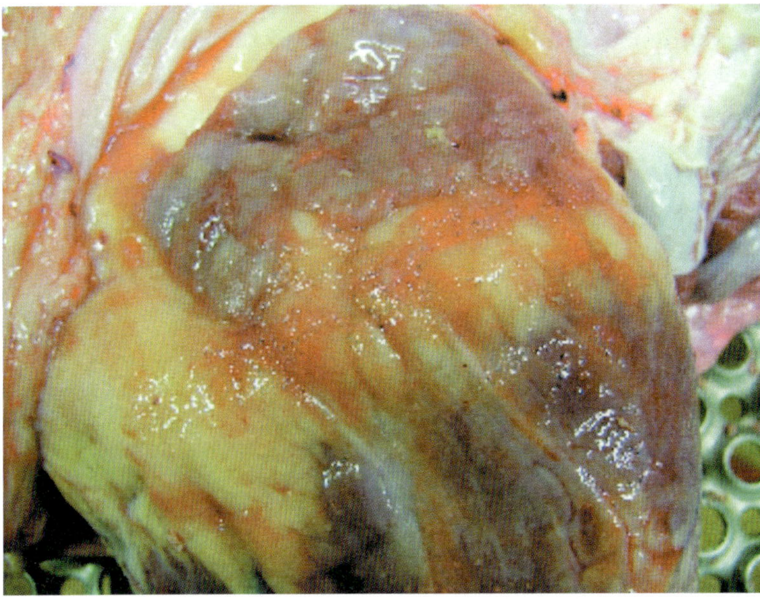

Epicarditis on a calf heart

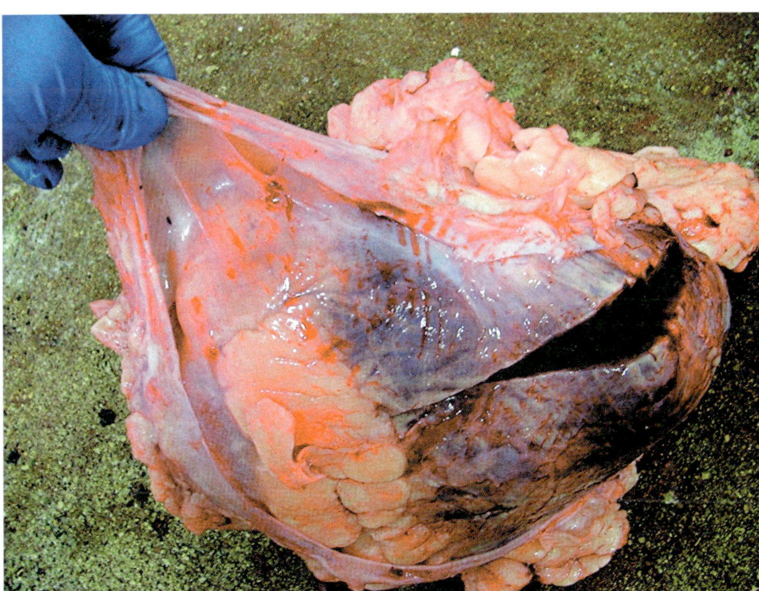

Pericarditis

Pericarditis in the bovine heart renders the organ unfit for human consumption. If the form of the pericarditis is acute and septic it can lead to rejection of the entire carcase and associated offal.

Endocarditis is the inflammation of the endocardium, the internal surface of the heart.

This condition is nearly always confined to the valves of the heart and tends to be bacterial in origin, normally involving bacterial strains such as Streptococci and *Corynebacterium pyogenes*. In cattle the tricuspid valve is most commonly affected.

Typical lesions observed range from pus plaques and ulcers to vegetative growths on the valves.

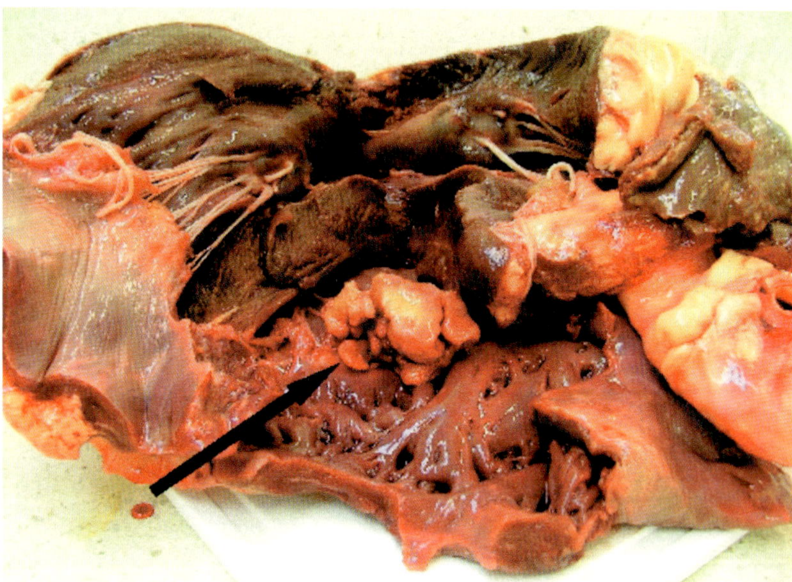

Vegetative endocarditis (arrowed) evident in this incised heart

In cases of endocarditis the heart is rejected as unfit for human consumption. The carcase is also inspected for signs of systemic infection, infarction of the kidneys and signs of septicaemia that could warrant rejection of the entire carcase and associated offal.

PERITONITIS

Peritonitis is inflammation of the peritoneum. The peritoneum is a membrane that lines the abdominal cavity and also covers the organs within that cavity. The part of the membrane lining the cavity is called the parietal peritoneum, that part covering the organs is called the visceral peritoneum.

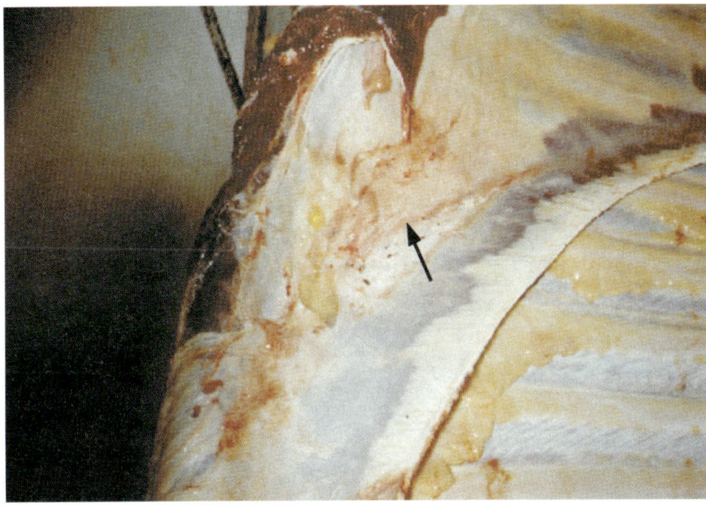

Parietal peritonitis

Peritonitis can be localised or diffuse, and can lead to adhesion of the peritoneum to organs and to itself.

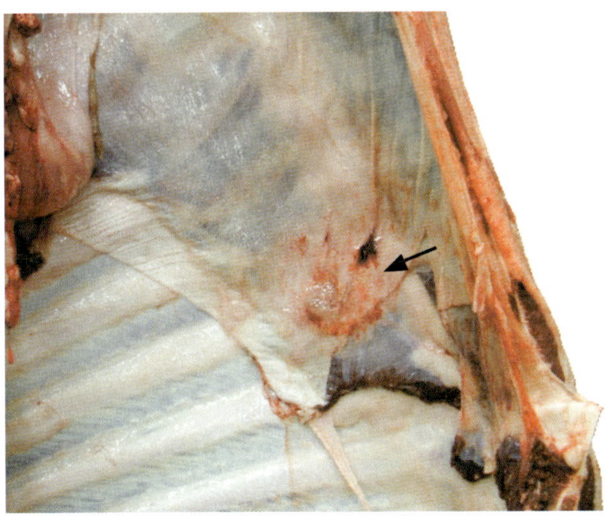

Parietal peritonitis

Chronic peritonitis can be produced by factors such as abscesses in the liver, and the affected parts are rejected.

Acute peritonitis is normally produced after bacterial infection of the membrane, either through a wound or as an infection from other areas, such as the stomach. Affected parts are rejected.

If the peritonitis becomes diffuse and septic the entire carcase and offal is rejected.

PLEURISY / PNEUMONIA

Pleurisy is inflammation of the pleura, a membrane that covers the lungs, heart and walls of the chest cavity. This can lead to the part of the lung adhering to the ribs and fluid build up. In the live animal breathing is painful, and the animal will tend to breathe using its' abdominal muscles rather than its ribcage. Pleurisy tends to be a complication of pneumonia.

If infected the pleura can be stripped from the ribs and rejected.

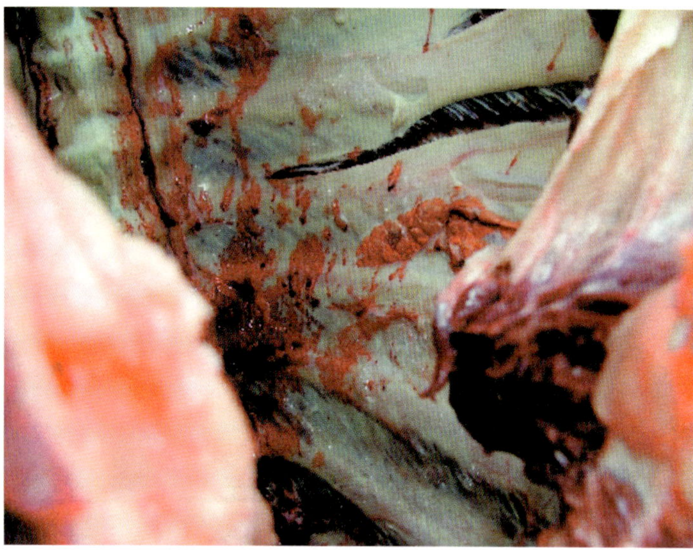

Parietal pleurisy

Pneumonia is best described as inflammation of the lung tissue itself. Viruses, bacteria, fungus, parasites etc can cause it.

There are two main types of pneumonia:

Broncho-pneumonia is characterised by small patches of pneumonia scattered among the normal lung tissue. This is an extension of a bronchial infection or due to blockage caused by parasites such as the lungworm *Dictyocaulus viviparus*.

Lobar pneumonia involves the whole or large part of a lung lobe. The lung tissue becomes consolidated and hepatised (liver like). There is a clear line of demarcation between affected tissue and the normal lung.

Both forms of pneumonia can become septic or gangrenous and may spread to the pleura. Septic pneumonia is fairly common, and the carcase is judged

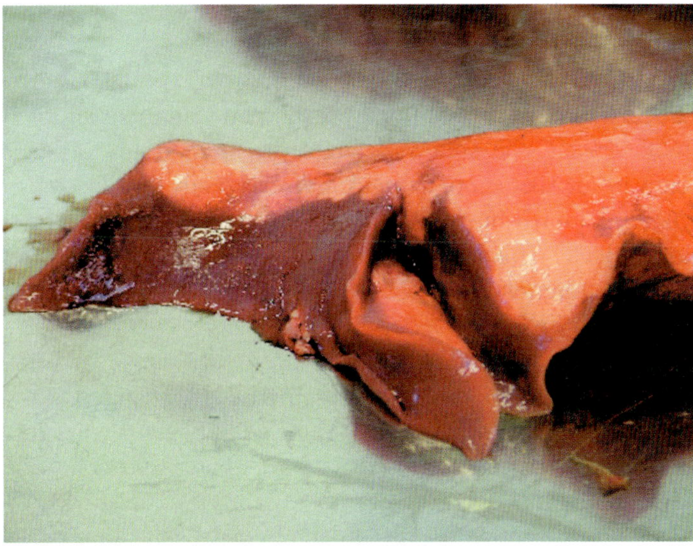

Hepatasized pneumonia – note obvious area of demarcation

on the evidence of systemic infection, if the evidence indicates a systemic infection the carcase and offal are rejected as unfit for human consumption.

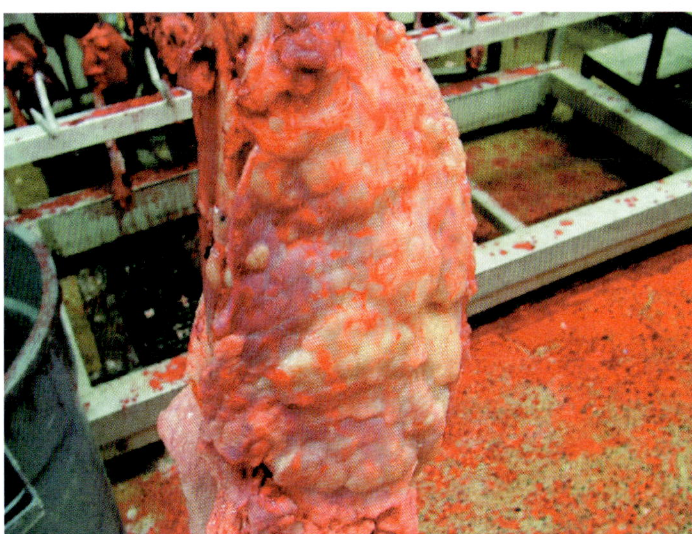

Lungs with pneumonia or pleurisy are rejected as unfit for human consumption

TELANGIECTASIS

Also known as cavernous haemangioma, angioma, 'plum pudding liver.'

A telangiectasia is a lesion formed by the expansion (dilation) of a group of small blood vessels; the area affected varies in size, up to 3mm.

This occurs in all species of animal, but especially in old cows. The liver substance contains bluish-black, spongy areas that are irregular in shape with clearly defined edges. This affection of the liver may vary from a few lesions, as normally seen in heifers and steers, to a generalised form found in mature cows.

Various theories have been proposed as to the cause of telangiectasis including bacterial infection and the stimulus of spinal nerves (as can occur during mating) causing dilation of the blood vessels supplying the liver. The latter theory is supported by the fact that the generalised condition tends to be an affection of mature cows.

Livers displaying minor areas of telangiectasis are trimmed; those with generalised telangiectasis are rejected as unfit for human consumption.

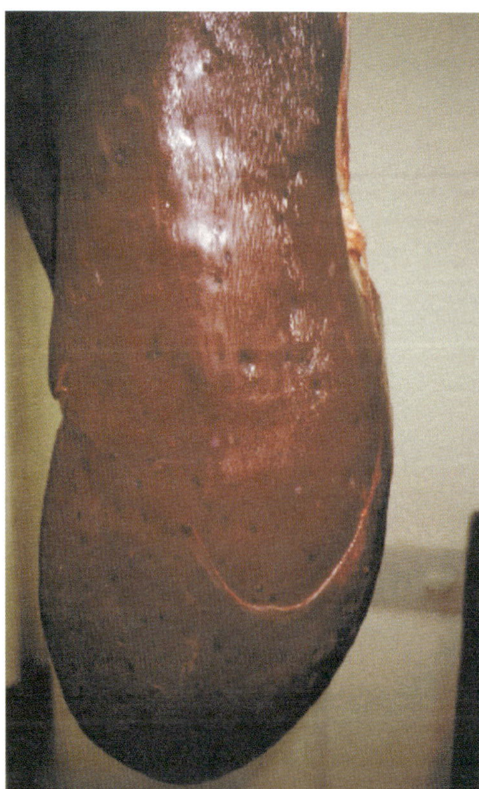

A typical 'plum pudding' liver

TRAUMA

The title trauma denotes any injury to the animal that warrants rejection of part or the entire carcase as unfit for human consumption. Any trauma to the animal pre-slaughter, i.e. before the blood is drained, can produce associated bruising (haemorrhage); all cases of pre slaughter trauma should be examined with a view to their welfare implications. These injuries can include:

Bone fractures – the local area is trimmed and rejected, due to both haemorrhage and the possibility of bone fragments. Depending on the age and condition of the fracture, the transportation of the affected animal may be in breach of Animal Welfare Legislation governing movement and transport and at the very least may raise welfare concerns. Fractures that occur after slaughter will not be associated with haemorrhage.

Split aitches – cattle are prone to splaying of the rear legs, causing fracture and/or bruising to the pelvic channel. Affected parts are trimmed and rejected.

Stick marks – These appear as red marks on the back, flank and hindquarters of the carcase and are subcutaneous haemorrhages (under skin bruising) caused by stick use in moving animals. Stick bruises are characterised by parallel lines of bruising with a central unhaemorrhagic area. Affected areas are trimmed and rejected.

Bruising – Can be caused by various means, often the lairaging of horned and unhorned cattle from different peer groups can lead to aggression and injury. Small areas of bruising are trimmed and rejected, although if this occurs in a large percentage of the batch it will be reported to the appropriate authorities.

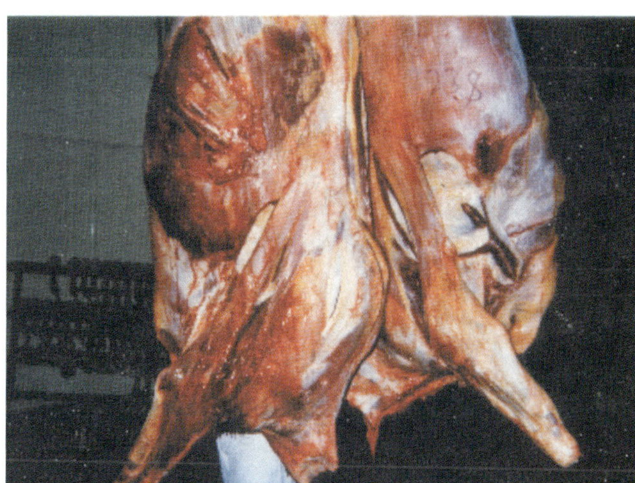

Horn damage

TRAUMATIC RETICULITIS

Also known as traumatic reticuloperitonitis, traumatic gastritis, 'hardware disease'.

This is a disease condition in cattle resulting from perforation of the part of the stomach (the reticulum) by a sharp object. This can occur as cattle do not completely chew their food, and the opening of the reticulum to the next stomach compartment (the omasum) is quite high allowing heavier metallic objects to remain in the reticulum. The honeycombed internal surface of the reticulum also promotes lodging of objects which then penetrate the wall of the reticulum during the contractions associated with rumination.

If the foreign object pierces the wall of the reticulum it can promote contamination of the peritoneal (abdominal) cavity. The bodies' immune response causes peritonitis (visceral and/or parietal), which can result in viscera adhering to surfaces, and also to septic peritonitis if gut bacteria are introduced into the cavity. The foreign object may also penetrate the diaphragm, setting up infection in the chest (thoracic) cavity, and the anatomical positioning of the reticulum in relation to the thoracic cavity also increases the opportunity for the membrane surrounding the heart (pericardium) to be pierced causing pericarditis and affecting the function of the heart.

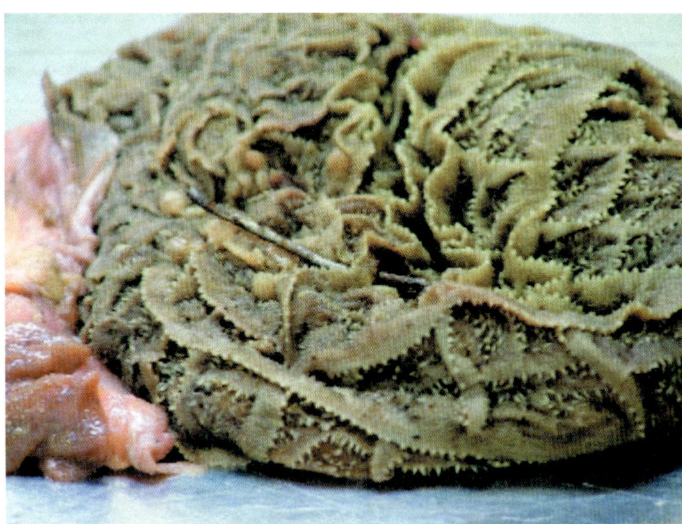

Wire protruding from the internal surface of the reticulum

A magnetic bolus is occasionally used by producers as a preventative measure. It remains in the reticulum and attracts any metallic objects ingested rendering a proportion of them safe. Examination of material found to cause traumatic reticulitis and occasional traumatic pericarditis in cattle would appear to indicate that the most prevalent form of wire encountered appears to be that used within car tyre walls, raising the hypothesis that the breakdown of tyres used as a sheet weighting system for silage heaps may introduce the wire into the feedstuff. Any infection created can remain localised, or can spread causing pyaemia or septicaemia to be set up.

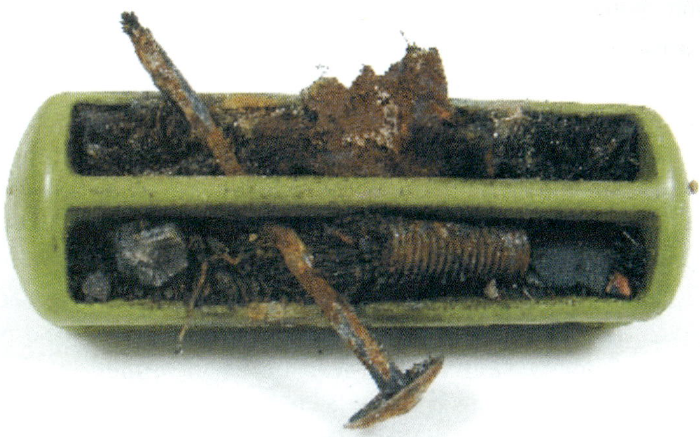

A magnetic bolus, illustrating material it attracts during the life of the beast

The affected areas are rejected, in severe cases where a systemic infection is evident the entire carcase and associated offal is rejected as unfit for human consumption.

TUBERCULOSIS

Tuberculosis is a chronic wasting disease of humans and animals caused by a tubercle bacillus, *Mycobacterium bovis* being the most predominant cause of the disease in cattle.

There are five ways the infection can gain entry to the body, these being by respiration (breathing), ingestion (swallowed), inoculation (injected), genital (during intercourse) and congenital. In calves the infection tends to be congenital, passed from the mother via the umbilicus before the calf is born.

The disease begins with a primary focus, in cattle this is normally in the lungs. Drainage from this leads to formation of lesions in adjacent lymph nodes. The initial lesion causes the formation of tumour-like masses (tubercles) by stimulating the body's immune response leading to the covering of the infected area with dense, fibrous tissue, the subsequent tubercle formation that normally prevents further spread of the infection. However if bacteria escape from this area they travel via the blood and lymph stream and lodge in other areas of the body causing further tubercles to be formed. As the tubercle grows the centre, deprived of nutrients, dies (necrosis) and solidifies due to mineralization.

In the acute form of the disease, large numbers of the bacilli gain entry into the body and form lesions containing large numbers of necrotic areas (foci) that resemble millet seed, thus giving the term miliary tuberculosis, a form of the disease that can be rapidly fatal.

Animals affected with tuberculosis become emaciated and further spread the infection amongst their peers, especially in the cases of lung lesions, which induce a hacking, constant coughing spreading the bacilli in aerosol form where it can be breathed in by other animals.

Due to the circulatory spread, tuberculous lesions in either form (tubercle or miliary) can be found in any organ. The classic, chronic tuberculosis of cattle involves the pleura (membrane of the chest cavity) or the peritoneum (lining of the stomach cavity). In these cases the tubercles form on the membranes in clusters giving rise to the term 'grapes' in the pleural cavity and 'pearl disease' in the peritoneal cavity.

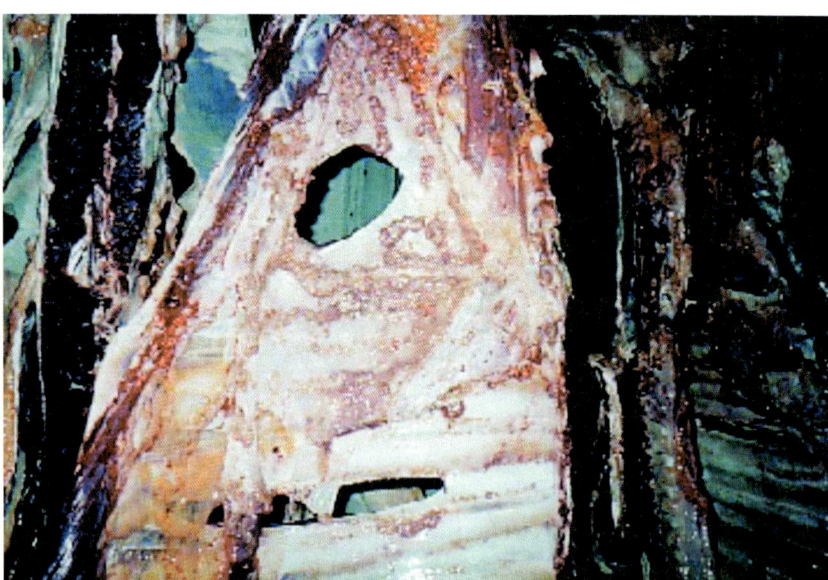

Tuberculosis in the peritoneum

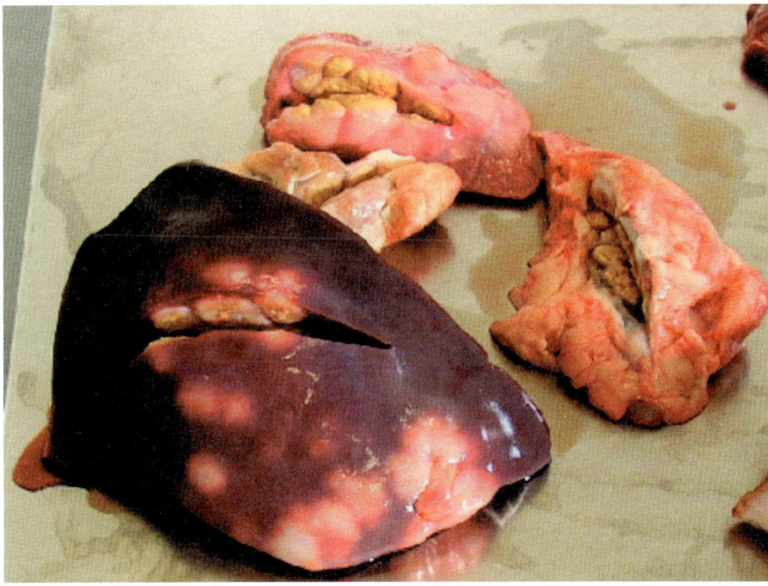

Tuberculous lesions in liver and lymph nodes

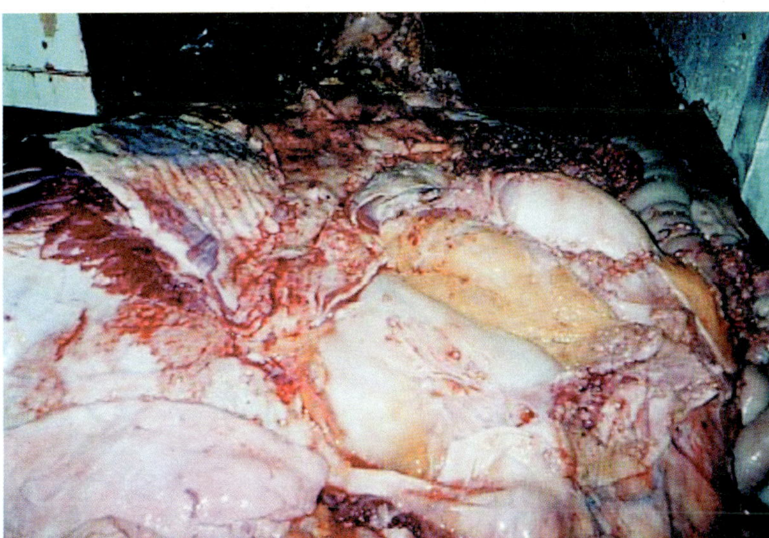

Tuberculosis lesions on the intestines and mesentery

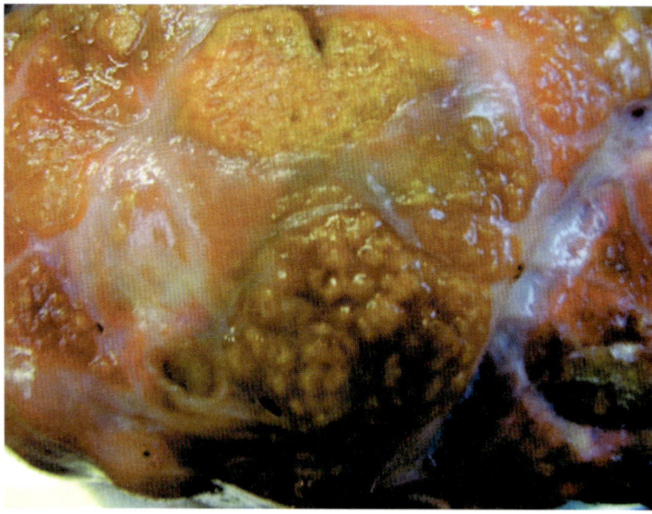

Tuberculous lesions in a bovine liver.

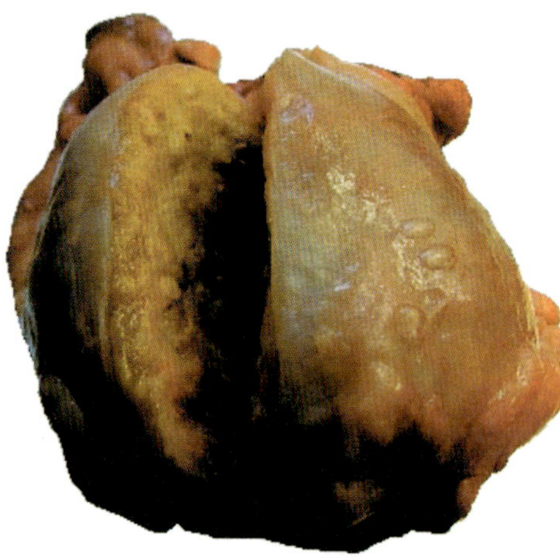

Tuberculosis in a mediastinal lymph node

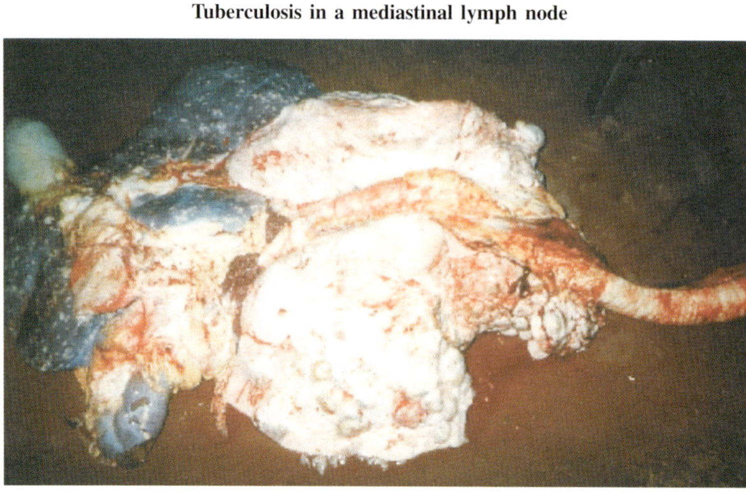

Miliary tuberculosis evident in this liver, tubercles in the lungs

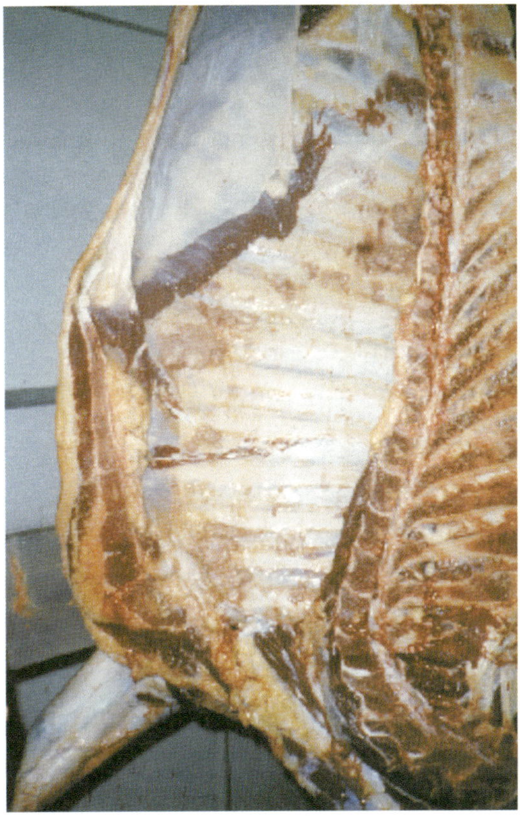

Tuberculous 'grapes' on the pleura

Carcases with generalised tuberculosis are rejected with their associated offal as unfit for human consumption.

URAEMIA

Uraemia is an affection where urine is absorbed into the circulating blood, normally as a result of obstruction of the normal flow of urine from the body.

Urine is a fluid containing water and the soluble waste products of the body. It is produced within the kidneys and flows down two ureters to the bladder, where it is stored until it is voided through the urethra. The waste products include urea and other nitrogen type products that are produced as a result of proteins and amino acid reactions in the body; these are filtered out in the kidneys.

Kidney (or renal) failure obstructs the normal flow of urine, as can occur in animals suffering from hydronephrosis or pyelonephritis. Other conditions such as urethritis (inflammation of the urethra), ureteroliths (stones in the ureters), and renal calculi (kidney stones) can also obstruct the flow of urine.

The reabsorbed waste which is carried by the blood to all the organs and tissues of the body gives the flesh a pronounced smell of urine, affecting the odour of the entire carcase and offal.

A quick test for uraemia in a carcase makes use of the fact that the smell of urine increases when the tissues are heated. A piece of muscle is removed from the carcase after 24 hours and boiled or fried. In cases of uraemia the smell increases. This is useful in determining whether the smell of urine is due to uraemia or the incision of the bladder during evisceration.

Carcases and their associated offal are rejected as unfit for human consumption in confirmed cases of uraemia.

XANTHOSIS

Xanthosis is thought to be a hereditary condition that causes a dark brown colouration of muscles due to a pigment xanthine.

This condition occurs in all breeds of cattle, but the Ayrshire breed is particularly susceptible, raising the theory that a genetic factor may be involved.

Most commonly affected are the heart, tongue and masseter (cheek) muscles, although any muscle may be affected. Generally, lymph nodes and glands near the kidneys (adrenal bodies) are enlarged and dark brown. The kidneys can also be affected.

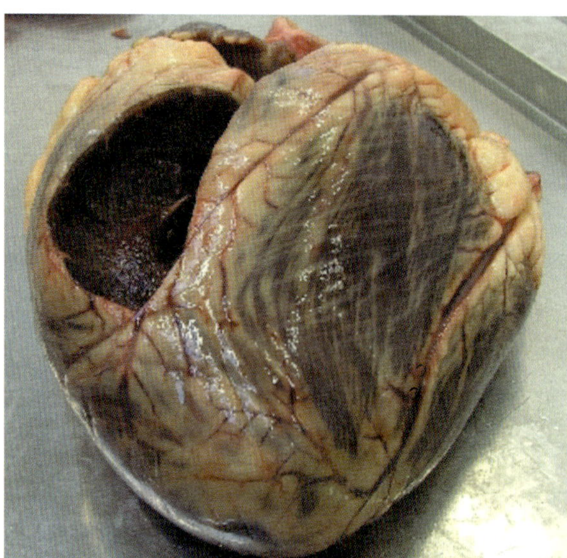

Xanthosis in a bovine heart

Affected parts are rejected as unfit for human consumption.

IMMATURITY

The flesh of immature animals is not permitted for human consumption. The determination of the age of a calf can obviously be achieved through the passport, but this is seldom available at the inspection point.

Factors that are taken into consideration at the inspection point include:

The state of the hooves; if they are soft, yellowish and the sole pads are convex it is a sign of lack of use and immaturity. This is termed 'Golden slippers.

The state of the umbilicus; the umbilical cord becomes dry and black after 4-5 days.

Atelectasis of the lungs; in an immature calf the lungs will be unexpanded and lung material will sink if placed in cool/cold water

The flesh is wet, usually greyish-red, is loose and flabby and can be easily torn with the fingers.

The fat around the kidneys is unformed, jelly-like and contains small particles of fat.

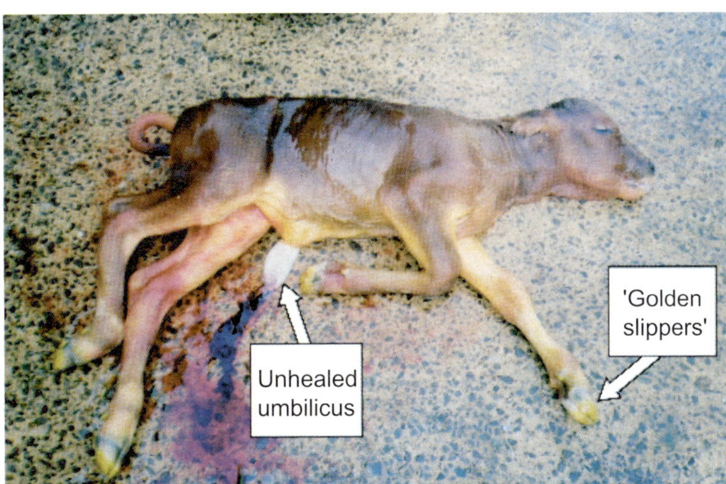

Immature carcases are rejected as unfit for human consumption

JOINT ILL

Joint ill is the term used to describe acute septic arthritis in calves. It originates from an umbilical infection and presents itself as an acute inflammation of the joints (especially the stifle) where the clear, lubricating synovial fluid becomes thickened and contains pus. If the inspector deems it necessary the joints can be incised to examine them for evidence of this.

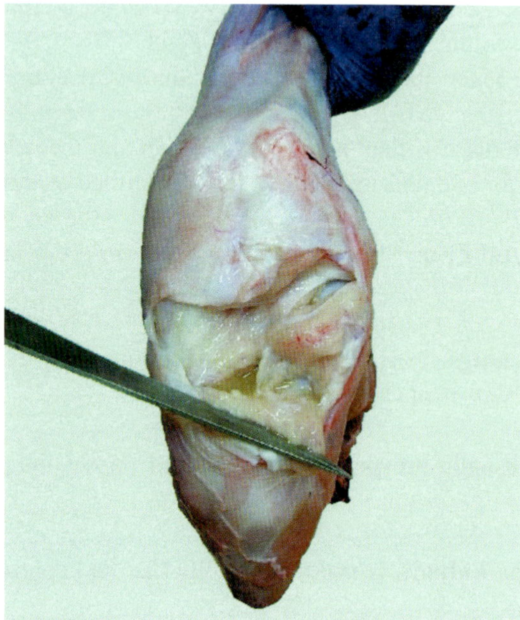

Joint ill – incision into a swollen hock joint revealing purulent synovial fluid

Calves with joint ill are rejected as unfit for human consumption.

WHARTON'S JELLY

An affection peculiar to calves is the deposition of sub capsular jelly-like fluid on the parietal surface of the liver usually near the falciform ligament. Wharton's jelly is the term given to an intracellular substance found in the foetal umbilicus; evidence suggests that this is a developmental cyst that regresses as it is seldom found in adult cattle.

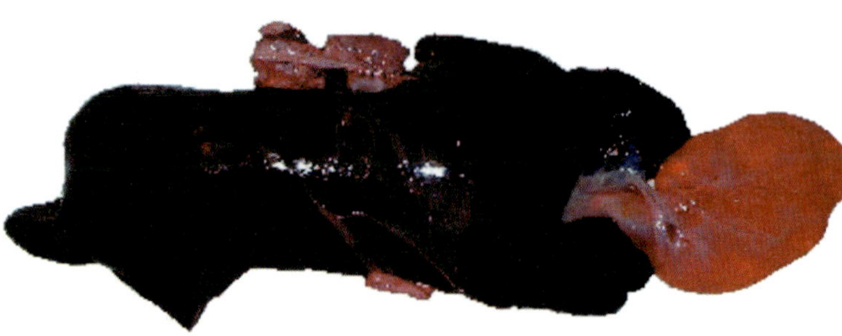

A calf liver with subcapsular 'Wharton's Jelly'

6

AIDE MEMOIRE - ANATOMY

Vertebral Column

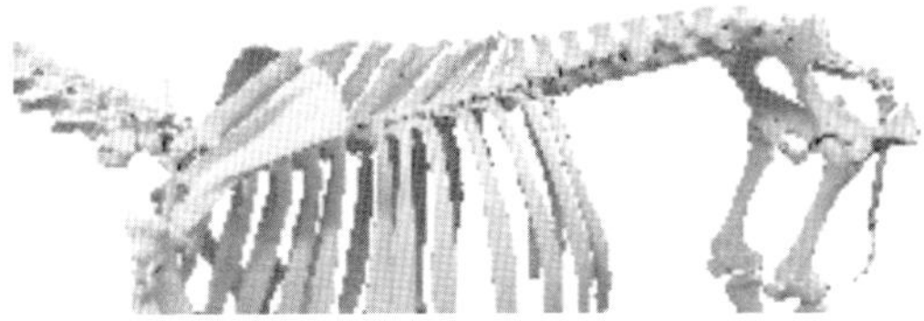

- 7 cervical vertebrae
- 13 thoracic vertebrae
- 6 lumbar vertebrae
- 5 sacral vertebrae
- 18-20 coccygeal vertebrae

Foreleg

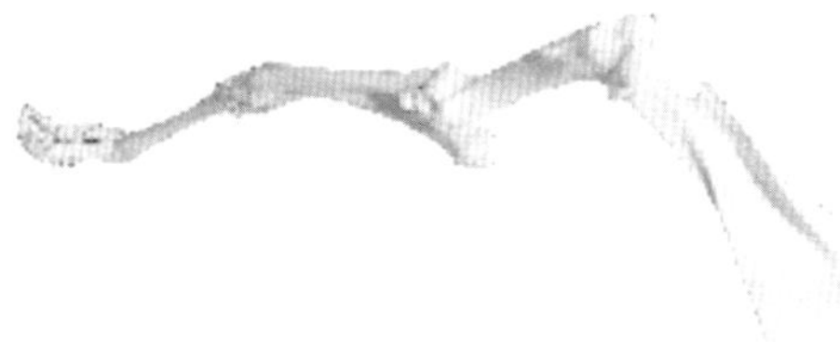

- Scapula
- Humerus
- Radius
- Ulna
- Carpus
- Metacarpus
- Phalanges

Hind Leg

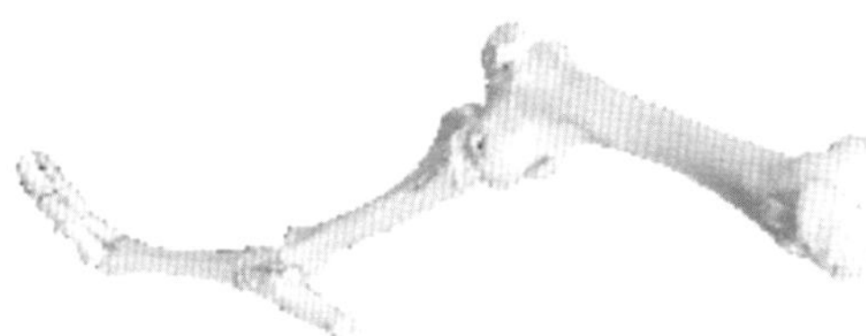

- Femur
- Patella
- Tibia
- Fibula
- Tarsus
- Metatarsus
- Phalanges
- Head of femur articulates with acetabulum of pelvis

Pelvis

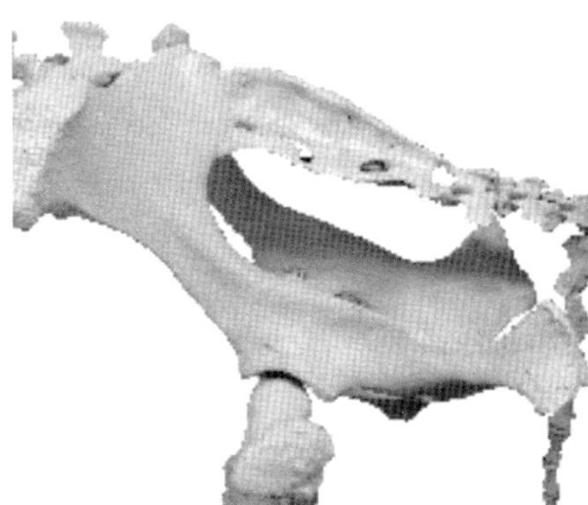

- 3 bones, ilium, ischium and pubis.
- Top of cavity formed by sacral vertebrae
- Paired pubis joined by pubic symphysis

Tongue

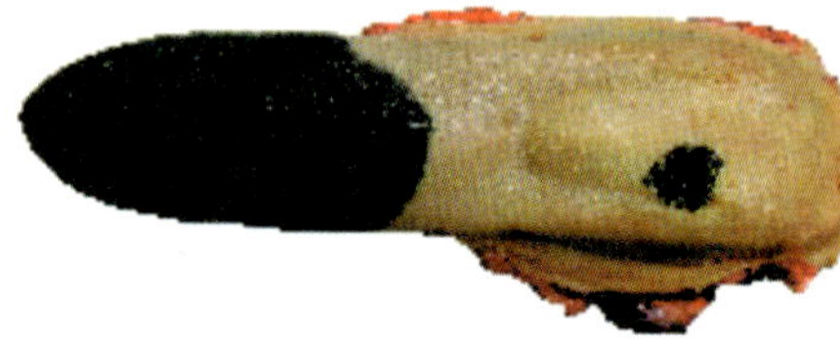

- Occasionally pigmented
- Dorsal prominence on upper surface
- Conical papillae on tip
- Fungiform papillae scattered on surface
- Lenticular papillae especially on dorsal prominence
- Vallate papillae grouped either side of dorsal prominence
- Weight Approx 1-1.25Kg Adult

Trachea / Lungs

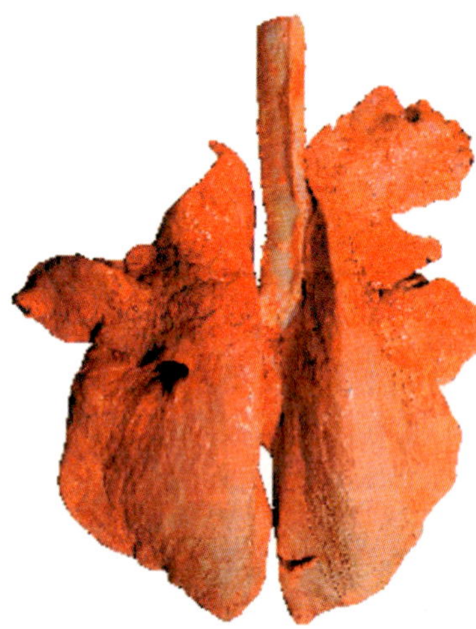

- Large bore trachea
- Approximately 50-55 cartilage rings
- Overlap of rings creates dorsal ridge
- 3 main bronchi, one to each lung and 1 accessory bronchus to right apical lobe
- Right lung has 4 lobes
  1 apical
  2 cardiac
  1 diaphragmatic
- Left lung has 3 lobes
  1 apical
  1 cardiac
  1 diaphragmatic
- Lungs covered by visceral pleura
- Weight Approx 2.5-3.5Kg adult

Heart

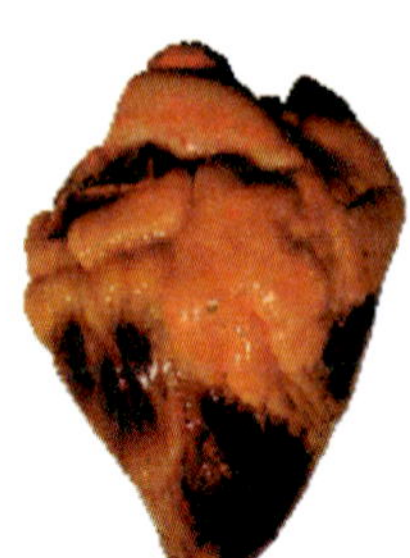

- Fat is crispy due to stearin
- 2 bones present at aortic origin
- 3 ventricular furrows
- 4 chambers, left atrium and ventricle, right atrium and ventricle.
- Average heartbeat 60-80 bpm at rest for adults, 100-120 bpm in calves.
- Weight approx. 2Kg adult

Spleen

- Flat and oval in outline
- Bluish/red in colour
- White Malphigian corpuscles visible in red pulp when incised
- Attached to rumen
- Weight approx. 1-1.5Kg adult

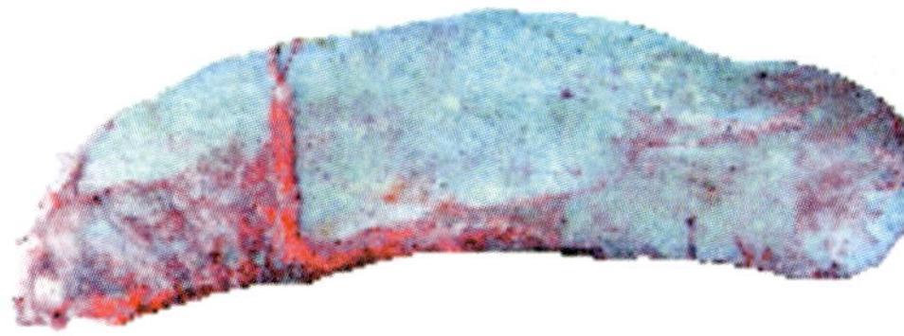

Kidneys

- Paired
- Right kidney held tight to body
- Left loose, more mobile
- 15-20 lobules
- Reddish brown in colour
- Left kidney rotated about its axis
- Weight 275-350g each in adults

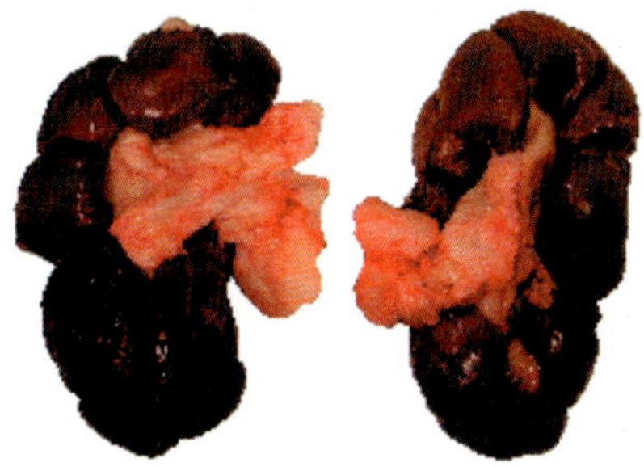

Rumen

- First stomach compartment
- Fermentation vessel, food moved in churning motion.
- Leaf-like papillae
- Protozoa and bacterial colonies present that act on ingesta
- Food bolus regurgitated and remasticated providing further mechanical breakdown and addition of saliva before re-entering rumen.

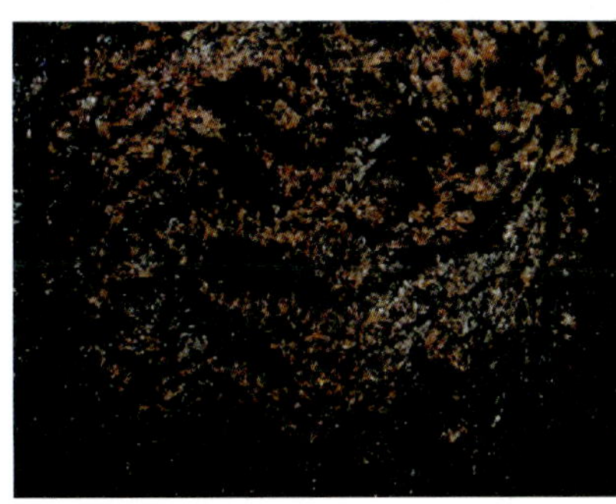

Reticulum

- Second stomach compartment
- Also known as the 'honeycomb'

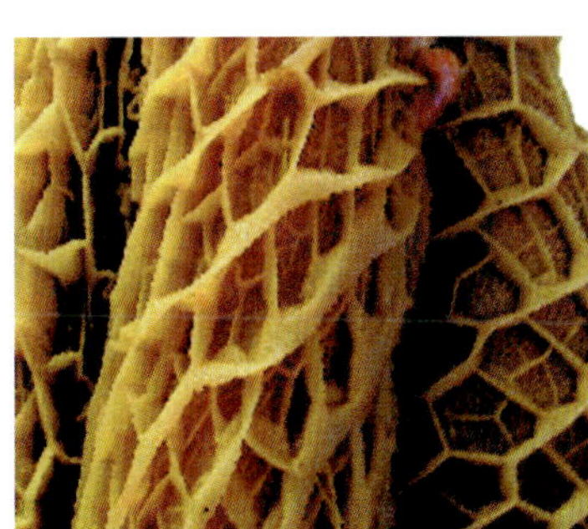

Omasum

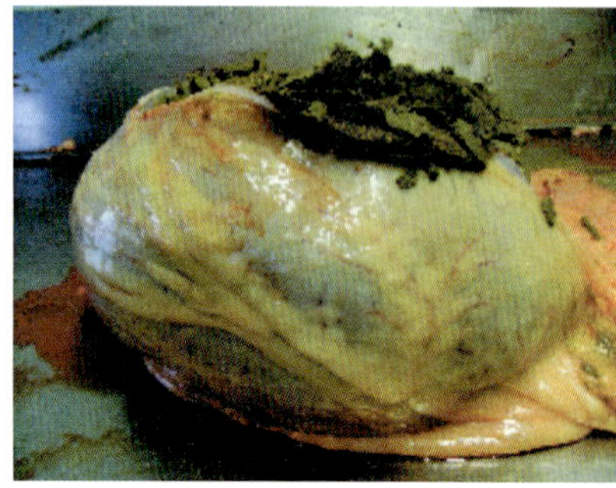

- Third stomach compartment
- Also known as 'manyplies', 'bible', 'psalterium'. Refers to tightly packed laminae.
- Ingesta forced between laminae and ground, smaller particles pass into abomasum

Abomasum

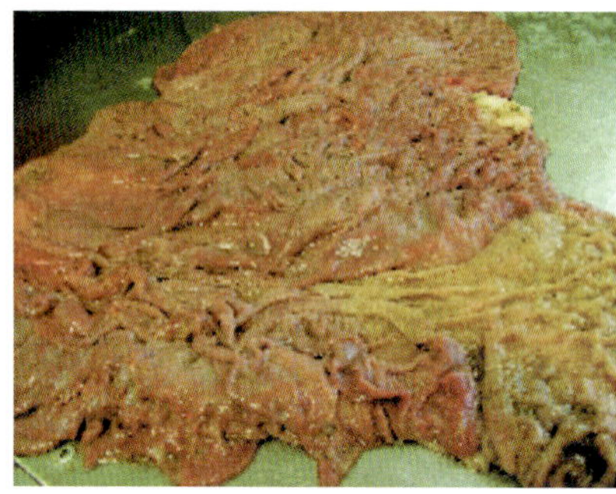

- True gastric stomach
- Glandular cells in mucosa secrete gastric juice.
- Also known as the reed in adults and the 'vell' in calves.

Liver

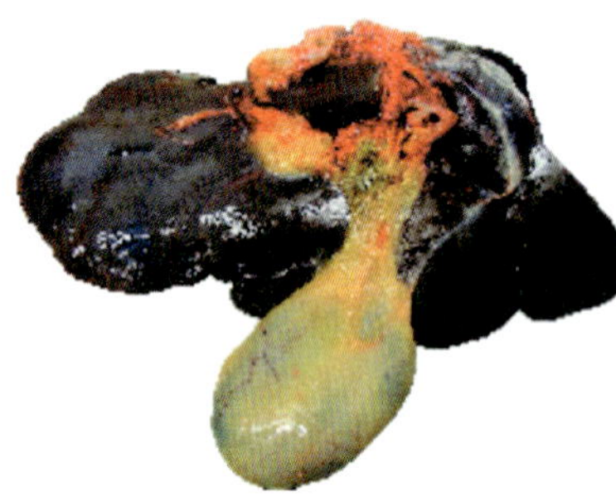

- 3 lobes, left, right and caudate lobe
- Pear shaped gall bladder
- Renal impression at base of caudate lobe.
- Umbilical groove on outer edge of left lobe.
- Hepatic lymph nodes surround portal opening
- Weight approx 5.5-6.5Kg adult

Uterus

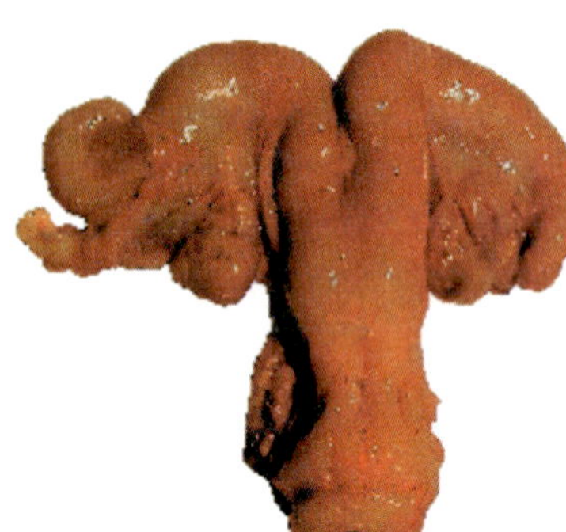

- Y-shaped muscular organ
- Size varies with age
- Two horns (cornua) lead to ovaries
- When horns are separated a double fold of the intercornual ligament is visible
- Ovaries appear cystic.
- Yellowish formation on ovaries follows release of ova into cornua.
- Muscular cervix separates uterus from vagina
- Uterus situated ventrally to rectum

Testicle

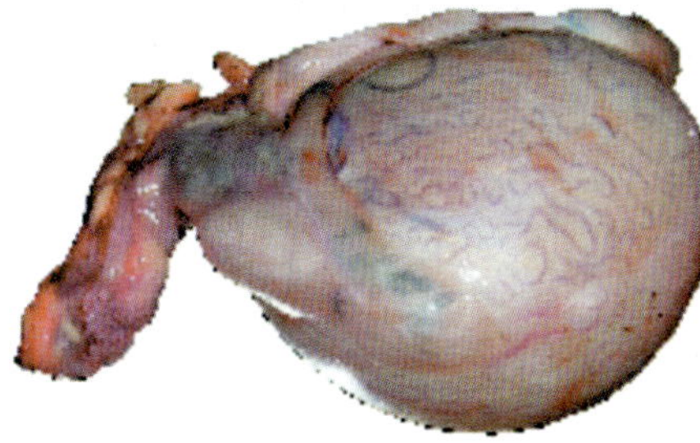

- Heavily veined and oval in shape.
- Prominent conical swelling at base formed by tail of epididymis.
- Epididymis leads to ductus deferens (vas deferens) that carries sperm to urethra.
- Internal surfaces yellowish and lobulated.
- Weight range 275-350g adult

7

DISEASE AND CAUSATIVE ORGANISM

DISEASE	CAUSE	TYPE
Actinobacillosis (Wooden Tongue)	*Actinobacillus ligniersi*	Bacterial
Actinomycosis (Lumpy jaw)	*Actinomyces bovis*	Bacterial
Anthrax (Woolsorters Disease, Splenic fever, Charbon, Malignant pustule)	*Bacillus anthracis*	Bacterial
Black Disease	*Clostridium novyi*	Bacterial
Blackleg	*Clostridium chauvoei*	Bacterial
Bovine Malignant Catarrh	Herpesvirus	Viral
Bovine Spongiform Encephalopathy (BSE, Mad Cow Disease)	Prion Protein	Prion
Bovine Virus Diarrhoea (BVD, Mucosal disease)	BVD virus, Pestivirus	Viral
Braxy (Bradsot)	*Clostridium septicum*	Bacterial
Brucellosis (Contagious abortion, Bangs disease, Undulant fever)	*Brucella abortus*	Bacterial
Calf Diphtheria (Oral necrobacillosis, necrotic stomatitis)	*Fusobacterium necrophorum*	Bacterial
Coccidiosis	*Eimeria bovis*	Protozoal
Contagious Bovine Pleuropneumonia	*Mycobacterium mycoides*	Bacterial
Contagious Bovine Pylelonephritis	*Corynebacterium renale*	Bacterial
Enzootic Bovine Leukosis (EBL, Bovine Viral Leukosis, Bovine Lymphosarcomas)	Retrovirus	Viral
Fascioliasis (Fluke)	*Fasciola hepatica*	Parasitic
Foot and Mouth Disease (FMD, Apthous fever)	Picornavirus	Viral

DISEASE	CAUSE	TYPE
Hydatidosis	*Echinococcus granulosus*	Parasitic
Infectious Keratoconjunctivitis (New Forest Disease, Pinkeye, Blight)	*Haemophilus bovis*	Bacterial
Infectious Rhinotracheitis (IBR, Red Nose)	Bovine Herpesvirus	Viral
Jöhne's Disease (Paratuberculosis)	*Mycobacterium paratuberculosis*	Bacterial
Leptospiridiosis	*Leptospira hardjo*	Bacterial
Listeriosis (Circling disease, Listerial meningocephalitis)	*Listeria monocytogenes*	Bacterial
Lungworm (Husk, Hoose, Parasitic Bronchitis)	*Dictyocaulus viviparus*	Parasitic
Ostertagiosis (Parasitic gastritis)	*Ostertagia ostertagi*	Parasitic
Papillomas (Warts)	Papilloma virus	Viral
Rabies (Hydrophobia, Lyssa)	Lyssa virus	Viral
Red Water Disease (Bacillary haemoglobinuria)	*Clostridium haemolyticum*	Bacterial
Red Water Fever (Cattle tick fever, Babesiosis)	*Babesia bovis* *Babesia divergens*	Protozoal
Ringworm	*Trichophyton verrucosum*	Fungal
Salmonellosis (Paratyphoid)	*Salmonella dublin*	Bacterial
Shipping Fever (Transit fever, Bovine Respiratory Disease)	*Pasteurella multocida* *Pasteurella haemolyticum*	Bacterial
Tenuicollis	*Taenia hydatigena*	Parasitic
Tetanus	*Clostridium tetani*	Bacterial
Tuberculosis (TB, Consumption)	*Mycobacterium bovis*	Bacterial

8

AFFECTIONS OF SPECIFIC PARTS

This section gives details of visible lesions and possible diagnosis, it is only intended as a guide

N.B. Neoplasia can affect all parts

LESION	POSSIBLE DIAGNOSIS
BONES	
Inflammation of	Osteitis
Purulent inflammation of	Osteomyelitis
Softening, swelling and curvature	Rickets (vitamin D deficiency)
Brown pigmentation	Osteohaematochromatosis
Tubercles (most common in vertebrae)	Tuberculosis
Callous formation	Resolving fracture,
HEAD	
Bones	
Swelling of mandible/ other bones	Actinomycosis, osteomyelitis, trauma
Brownish red discolouration	Osteohaematochromatosis
Buccal cavity	
Inflammation of	Stomatitis
Erosion of mucous membrane	Bovine Virus Diarrhoea, Foot and mouth
Necrotic areas on pharynx	Calf diphtheria, traumatic infection
Diphtheric foul smelling membrane	Calf diphtheria
Crater like erosions of nose, mouth	Malignant catarrhal fever
Erosion of cheek papillae	Trauma, Malignant catarrhal fever
Eyes	
Ulceration of cornea	Infectious Keratoconjunctivitis, trauma
Opaque cornea	Malignant catarrhal fever, Infectious Keratoconjunctivitis
Conjunctivitis	Injury, Malignant catarrhal fever, Infectious Keratoconjunctivitis
Cataracts in calves	Bovine virus diarrhoea,
Lymph nodes	
Necrotic/caseous/calcified lesions	Actinomycosis, Tuberculosis, Abscess
Muscle	
Pea sized cyst (can be calcified/caseated) single scolex	*Cysticercus bovis*
Black 'ink splashes'	Melanosis
Brown discolouration	Xanthosis
Skin	
Warts	Papilloma virus, Papillomas (neoplasia)
Scabby, scaly, loss of hair	Ringworm, mange, rubbing damage

LESION	POSSIBLE DIAGNOSIS
HEART	
Inflammation of pericardium	Pericarditis
Inflammation of heart surface	Epicarditis
Inflammation of heart muscle	Myocarditis
Inflammation of internal structures	Endocarditis
Longitudinal yellowish/white bands	Foot and Mouth Disease
Haemorrhages	Septicaemia, toxaemia, Salmonellosis, Contagious Bovine Pleuropneumonia, toxaemia, septicaemia
Opaque serous membrane	Pericarditis (traumatic, fibrinous or septic)
Brown discolouration	Xanthosis
Black 'ink splashes'	Melanosis
Yellow fat	Jaundice, carotene pigmentation, xanthrophyll pigmentation
Necrotic areas	Listeriosis
Pea sized cyst (can be calcified/caseated) single scolex	*Cysticercus bovis*
Tumours	Sporadic leukosis, Enzootic Bovine Leukosis
Cauliflower like growths on heart valves	Vegetative endocarditis
Fluid filled cysts containing 'sand'	Hydatid cyst
INTESTINES	
Inflammation of	Enteritis
Tiger stripes in colon	Malignant catarrhal fever
Oedema and petechial haemorrhage	Malignant catarrhal fever, toxaemia, Salmonellosis
Crater like erosion of intestinal mucosa	Malignant catarrhal fever
Ulcerative enteritis	Infectious bovine rhinotracheitis
Striped appearance of caecum and colon	Bovine virus diarrhoea
Sub mucosal Haemorrhage	Non specific enteritis, bovine virus diarrhoea
Thickened and corrugated mucosa	Jöhne's disease, toxins,
Haemorrhagic enteritis	(Severe) anthrax, Salmonellosis
Necrotic enteritis	Salmonellosis, listeriosis
JOINTS	
Inflammation of	Arthritis
Fluid filled cysts becoming fibrous over limb joints (Hygromas)	Trauma, pressure swellings, brucellosis

LESION	POSSIBLE DIAGNOSIS
KIDNEYS	
Inflammation of	Nephritis
White patches	Malignant catarrhal fever
Interstitial nephritis	Leptospiridiosis
White patches, pyramidal in section	Infarcts
Fatty degeneration	Enterotoxaemia, septicaemia
Crystalline 'balls' or stones	Renal calculi
Slimy fluid in renal pelvis	Pyelonephritis
Enlarged and fluid filled	Hydronephrosis, retention cysts, blockage of ureter
White/yellow raised foci	Fibroplastic nephritis in calves, tuberculosis, abscessation
Dark brown/black colouration	Xanthosis
LARYNX	
Inflammation of	Laryngitis
Acute inflammation	Infectious bovine rhinotracheitis
Erosions	Bovine virus diarrhoea
LIVER	
Inflammation of	Hepatitis
Fluke	Fascioliasis
Distended bile ducts	Fascioliasis, cholecystitis
Focal depressed bluish black spots throughout liver substance	Telangiectasis
Abscesses	Abscesses
Liver tissue replaced by fibrous tissue	Cirrhosis
Fluid filled cyst(s) containing 'sand' in liver tissue	Hydatidosis
Fluid filled sac on liver surface containing single white scolex	Tenuicollis
Black 'ink splashes'	Melanosis
Small pale necrotic foci in liver tissue	Bacterial necrosis, military tuberculosis
Liver is greasy and is friable to the touch	Fatty change, septicaemia/toxaemia
Nodules containing yellow pus - granular	Actinobacillosis, Tuberculosis
Nodules containing yellow pus - smooth	Tuberculosis, Actinobacillosis
Lymphoid growths in liver	Tumours, Enzootic Bovine Leukosis
Adhesion between liver and skirt, or alimentary tract	Peritonitis, traumatic peritonitis
Enlargement	Hepatitis, babesiosis
Reddish patches throughout substance	Haemangioma

LESION	POSSIBLE DIAGNOSIS
LUNGS	
Inflammation of lung tissue	Pneumonia
Inflammation of bronchi	Bronchitis
Inflammation of lung surface	Pleurisy, pleuritis
Acute inflammation of bronchi	Infectious bovine rhinotracheitis, bronchitis
Air bubbles visible between lung septa	Emphysema, Infectious bovine rhinotracheitis
Fibrinous pleurisy	Contagious bovine pleuropneumonia
Large area of lung or lobe hepatised or consolidated, well demarcated	Lobar pneumonia, Contagious bovine pleuropneumonia, shipping fever, lungworm, foreign body, Infectious bovine rhinotracheitis
Small areas of pneumonia	Broncho-pneumonia, aspiration pneumonia
Thread-like pieces in bronchi	Lungworm
Firm masses in lung tissue	Abscesses, tuberculosis, hydatid cysts
Fluid filled cysts	Hydatid cysts
Black 'ink splashes' in substance	Melanosis
MAMMARY GLANDS	
Inflammation of	Mastitis
Pale greenish/yellow abscesses	Corynebacterium pyogenes mastitis
Lymphoid masses	Neoplasia
Vesicles on teats	Cow pox, Foot and Mouth, trauma,
Udder swollen and hot, oedematous L.N.	Septic mastitis
Violet red to greenish black tissue	Gangrene
MUSCLE	
Brownish discolouration	Xanthosis
Localised fibrosis	Interstitial fibrosis, muscular fibrosis, post traumatic scarring
Fatty change	Steatosis, resolving traumatic injury
Pea sized cysts (can be calcified/viable)	*Cysticercus bovis*
Greenish foci in muscle fibres	Eosinophilic myositis
Jelly-like blood tinged infiltration	Resolving bruise
Swellings containing gas, discoloured serum	Blackleg, malignant oedema
1cm long greenish white oval cysts	Sarcocysts
OESOPHAGUS	
Granulomatous lesions in lower portion	Actinobacillosis, tuberculosis
Longitudinal shallow erosion	Malignant Catarrhal Fever
Inflammation of	Oesophagitis

LESION	POSSIBLE DIAGNOSIS
SKIN	
Inflammation of	Dermatitis
Circumscribed elevated patches, scaly or scabby	Rubbing injury, ringworm
Denuded areas	Rubbing injury, ringworm, mange
Cauliflower-like outgrowths	Papillomas
Subcutaneous nodules	Warble larvae (on back), skin tuberculosis
Erosion of skin/mucous membrane junction	Bovine virus diarrhoea
Vesicles/ulceration of coronary band of foot	Foot and Mouth Disease, Bovine virus diarrhoea
SPLEEN	
Inflammation of	Splenitis
Gross enlargement (splenomegaly)	Anthrax, mounting damage, babesiosis, bovine leucosis, septicaemia, 'slaughter spleen'
Granular nodules	Tuberculosis, abscesses, Actinomycosis
Cysts containing 'sand'	Hydatid cysts
Necrotic foci	Listeriosis
STOMACHS	
Inflammation of	Gastritis
Grossly distended rumen	Bloat, overfeeding
Inflammation of the abomasum	Ostertagiosis, poisoning
Nodules on gastric surface of abomasum	Ostertagiosis
Ulcerative lesions on pillars of rumen	Foot and mouth
Swollen and reddened abomasal folds	Malignant catarrhal fever
Ulceration and congestion of rumen	Bovine Virus diarrhoea
Ulceration of abomasal mucosa	Trauma, Leptospiridiosis
Haemorrhagic mucosa of abomasum	Trauma, gastritis, Leptospiridiosis, toxins, Salmonellosis
Raised plaques in mucosa - rumen	Actinobacillosis
Raised plaques in mucosa - reticulum	Actinobacillosis
TESTICLES	
Inflammation of	Orchitis
Abscessation of testes, spermatic cord	Brucellosis, traumatic infection
THORAX AND PLEURA	
Inflammation of pleura	Pleurisy, pleuritis
Hydrothorax, straw coloured	Contagious bovine pleuropneumonia
Adhesion	Parietal pleurisy

LESION	POSSIBLE DIAGNOSIS
THORAX AND PLEURA (contd)	
Lumps on ribs	Resolving fractures, lymphosarcomas
Tubercles, 'grapes'	Pleural tuberculosis
TONGUE	
Inflammation of	Glossitis
Nodules in substance	Actinobacillosis, injury, abscessation
Solid areas in tongue	Actinobacillosis, traumatic scar tissue
Erosion of conical papillae	Bovine Malignant Catarrh
Ulceration of mucosa, white epithelium	Foot and Mouth Disease, Bovine Virus Diarrhoea
Diphtheric membrane and foul smell	Calf diphtheria
Vesicles	Foot and Mouth Disease
TRACHEA	
Inflammation of	Tracheitis
Acute inflammation	Non-specific tracheitis, injury, infectious bovine rhinotracheitis
UTERUS	
Inflammation of	Metritis
Serous yellow/red to brown discharge	Septic metritis, brucellosis, retained placenta
Gross enlargement, foul odour, brownish pus	Septic metritis
Pustules in mucosa	Infectious bovine rhinotracheitis

INDEX

INDEX

A

B

C

D

E

F

G

H

I

J

K

L

M

N

O

P

R

U

V

W

X

Z